MUMS SHAPE UP

LISA WESTLAKE

WITH PHOTOGRAPHY BY BRONWYN KIDD

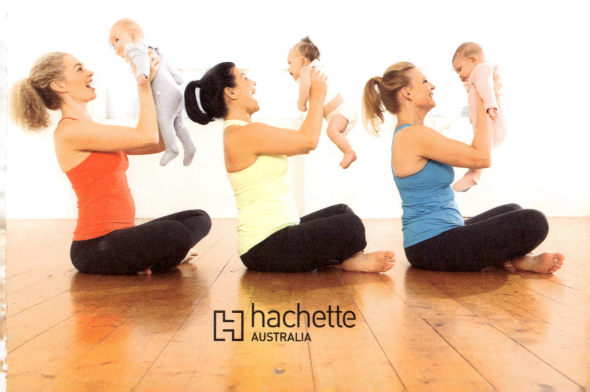

hachette
AUSTRALIA

AN IMPORTANT NOTE
The exercises in this book are designed as low-intensity, low-impact programs suitable for most postnatal women. If you have a history of certain medical conditions, including poorly controlled diabetes, high blood pressure and heart disease, you will need to be careful. Before undertaking any postnatal exercises, programs or classes always consult your doctor and only commence exercising that is compatible with your particular health situation and needs with their consent. Although every effort has been made to ensure that the contents of this book are accurate, it must not be treated as a substitute for qualified medical advice. To minimise the risk of incident/injury carefully read the information in parts one and two of this book, which contain critical information on important health considerations and safe exercising guidelines. Neither the author nor the publisher can be held responsible for any loss or claim arising out of the use, or misuse, of the suggestions made or the failure to take medical advice.

hachette
AUSTRALIA

Published in Australia and New Zealand in 2012
by Hachette Australia
(an imprint of Hachette Australia Pty Limited)
Level 17, 207 Kent Street, Sydney NSW 2000
www.hachette.com.au

10 9 8 7 6 5 4 3 2 1

Copyright © Lisa Westlake 2012

This book is copyright. Apart from any fair dealing for the purposes of private study, research, criticism or review permitted under the *Copyright Act 1968*, no part may be stored or reproduced by any process without prior written permission. Enquiries should be made to the publisher.

National Library of Australia
Cataloguing-in-Publication data:

Westlake, Lisa.
Mums shape up/Lisa Westlake.
978 0 7336 2835 1 (pbk)
Postnatal exercise.
Physical fitness for women.
Mothers–Health and hygiene.
Mothers.

613.7045

Photography by Bronwyn Kidd
Cover design by Christabella Designs
Text design by Agave Creative Group
Typeset in Avenir by Agave Creative Group
Printed in China by South China Printing Co. Ltd.

Hachette Australia's policy is to use papers that are natural, renewable and recyclable products and made from wood grown in sustainable forests. The logging and manufacturing processes are expected to conform to the environmental regulations of the country of origin.

Author's Note

The early days, weeks and months of motherhood are precious and exciting. Never is there a more important time for women to nurture and look after themselves, both physically and emotionally.

As a new mum, it is natural to want to get your body back in shape, but it is essential to take your time and exercise wisely. While postnatal exercise has many benefits, too much, too soon will hinder your recuperation and leave you vulnerable to unwanted short- and long-term problems so a gradual and sensible return to exercise as you bond with your new baby is the best approach.

I am delighted to follow up *Exercising for Two*, the safe and easy prenatal fitness guide, with its postnatal partner, *Mums Shape Up*, a sensible and effective approach to shaping up and feeling fantastic after having your baby. The books draw on my knowledge from over 20 years' instructing physiotherapy, pre- and postnatal fitness classes and unite a sound theoretical basis for postnatal recovery and fitness with practical applications and exercises to suit you and your new lifestyle. This book also recaps a few important prenatal fitness considerations so, together, we can move on to understanding postnatal changes and their exercise implications. A range of exercises and programs are included to assist you in designing your own fitness plan that will help you shape up and feel fantastic, while you enjoy motherhood.

A step-by-step recovery and return to fitness to help you manage the demands and enjoy the delights of early motherhood

contents

Congratulations   6
How to use this book   7
Preparing for labour and the early days of motherhood   8
The benefits of postnatal exercise   10

PART ONE – BEFORE YOU START

Pregnancy, labour and delivery   14
Looking after yourself, as well as your baby   16
Realistic goals and time frames   17
Fatigue, sleep and energy levels   20
Mood and morale   22
Breastfeeding   25
Nutrition and hydration   26
Extra-special thought   28
Pelvic floor first   29
Exercise and your pelvic floor   30
The ins and outs of abdominals   33
Engage your core   34
Posture and back health   38
Postnatal exercise guidelines   42
The early days   44
Early weeks   46
As the weeks turn to months   47

PART TWO – THE EXERCISES

Optimise your recovery and return to fitness 50
Mobility 52
Posture, core and pelvic floor 62
Cardiovascular fitness 82
Water fitness 92
At the gym 94
Strengthen and tone 96
Stroller fitness 138
Mum-and-bub workout 151
Relaxation 168
Stretching 170
Stretches 172

PART THREE – THE EXERCISE PROGRAMS

Exercise programs 180
Thank you 189

congratulations

Having picked up this book it is likely you are preparing for or have recently been through one of the most treasured experiences of your life; the arrival of your new baby. This is the time to optimise your physical and emotional well-being as you recover, regain your fitness and settle into being a new mum.

Nurturing your body and soul is as important now as it was during pregnancy. While you may feel focused on looking after your baby, you need to take care of yourself too. A healthy balance of rest, a nutritious diet and the right kinds of exercise will help you flourish and give you more energy to enjoy your new child.

Although many women are keen to get back in shape after the birth, too much, too soon can be detrimental to your recovery and lead to long-term problems. I therefore advise a gradual approach that will help you regain your waist, muscle tone and fitness without putting undue stress on your body and energy levels. The early days and weeks are a time for recovery, bonding and settling into your new role; be kind to yourself and patient with your body.

Mums Shape Up will help you understand your body's individual needs as you recover from pregnancy and labour and adapt to breastfeeding and the lifestyle of a new mother, guiding you towards appropriate exercise choices to help you get back in shape. Appreciating the physical and emotional demands of the child-bearing years will allow you to choose your exercises wisely, progress gradually and reap the benefits of a personalised postnatal fitness program.

How to use this book

Part One – Before you start
Focuses on the physical and emotional considerations of the early weeks and months of motherhood and explains their exercise implications with guidelines for sensible selection and progression.

Part Two – The exercises
Outlines a range of exercises to assist at all stages of postnatal fitness.

Part Three – The exercise programs
Every mother is unique. Select one of the 14 physiotherapy-designed fitness plans in this section to suit your goals, lifestyle and fitness level. Early motherhood is a precious time, but it can also be a challenging one. Sensible exercise, without overdoing it, can improve your physical and emotional fitness, helping you feel strong for your incredible new role.

As a physiotherapist I encourage you to be patient, focusing on recovery, health and well-being over weight-loss or appearance. Quality of exercise is more important than quantity.

As a fitness instructor I hope you will enjoy the benefits of a gradual return to exercise. Every day is different, so listen to your body.

As a mum, I say congratulations, trust your instincts and enjoy this precious time.

Lisa Westlake

Preparing for labour and the early days of motherhood

Exercising for two

Mums Shape Up is the postnatal companion to *Exercising for Two*, a comprehensive guide to prenatal exercise. Prenatal exercise has many benefits, including helping maintain fitness and strength as well as a happy, healthy state of mind. It also helps you to prepare physically and emotionally for labour and prepares you for recovery after your baby has arrived. It is important to ensure that your prenatal fitness program suits your fitness level and stage of pregnancy and is further modified if you experience pregnancy-related conditions such as back ache or pelvic-joint pain. The following points outline a few key prenatal fitness considerations that are covered in more detail in *Exercising for Two*.

You are unique Your fitness, stage of pregnancy and any medical conditions must be considered when designing your personal prenatal fitness plan. Check with your doctor or women's health physiotherapist before and throughout your pregnancy that your exercise program is safe and appropriate for you.

Look after your pelvic floor There is significant load on the pelvic floor during pregnancy and delivery so to keep it strong and help prevent incontinence and prolapse avoid high-impact exercise, heavy lifting and straining, and make pelvic-floor exercises a part of your daily routine.

Avoid strain on your joints Avoid overloading your joints – already vulnerable due to the hormones and added weight of pregnancy – keeping your movements smooth and controlled and focusing on core stability and good posture.

Modify your positions Lying on your back to exercise is not recommended after 16 weeks gestation, you will prefer positions other than horizontal if you experience reflux, and if you have carpal tunnel syndrome you should seek alternatives to exercises where you are weight-bearing through your hands. If you experience pelvic-joint discomfort, seek advice from a physiotherapist as you will need to modify your exercise style and positioning significantly.

Focus on your core Overworking the abdominals during pregnancy may lead to increased risk of abdominal separation (page 36). Focus instead on strengthening your deep, core abdominals.

Moderate exercise intensity Exercising three to four times a week at a mild to moderate intensity is ideal during pregnancy. Avoid over-exerting yourself, stay well-hydrated and cool, and do not exercise in hot environments.

Prepare for labour Practising labour preparation and relaxation exercises such as those in *Exercising for Two* will help you prepare physically and emotionally for labour.

Sensible exercise, a healthy diet and a positive attitude help you prepare for labour and early motherhood

The benefits of postnatal exercise

Sensible and appropriate exercise after having your baby has many benefits. It:

- helps you to recover after pregnancy, labour and delivery;
- allows you to return gradually to pre-pregnancy activities;
- prioritises recovery of important muscles affected by pregnancy, such as pelvic floor and abdominals, and helps them regain their pre-pregnancy strength and function;
- assists you to achieve and maintain a healthy body weight;
- boosts your general fitness, stamina and energy levels;
- enhances muscle tone, strength and definition;
- encourages healthy posture to combat the stresses on your body related to the life of a new mum;
- assists in prevention of postnatal problems such as incontinence and back pain;
- improves your quality of sleep;
- reduces anxiety and stress;
- enhances mood, morale and self-esteem;
- ensures designated time for you;
- provides social and emotional support (thanks to being around others, especially other new mums).

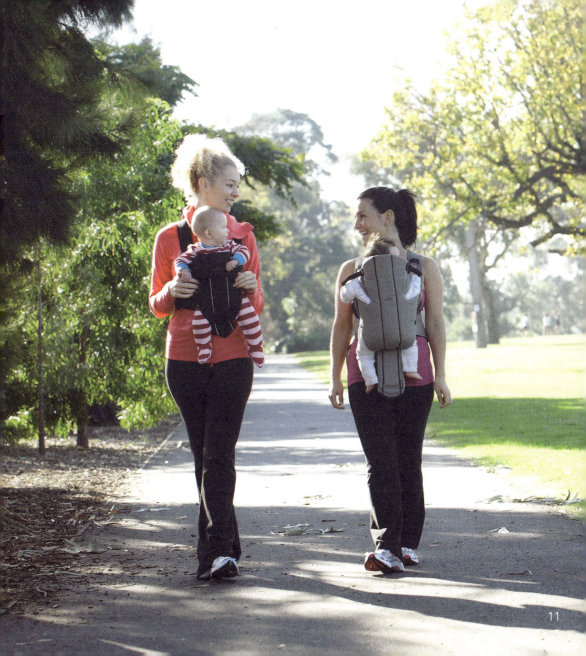

Know your body, look after your body

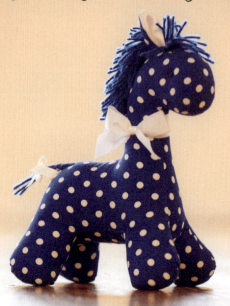
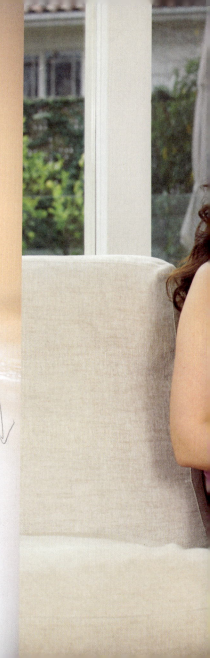

Several factors impact your ability to return to activity and exercise after your baby's delivery – your prior fitness, pregnancy, labour and delivery as well as your postnatal situation must all be taken into account. Understanding how they affect your ability to exercise will enable you to make wise fitness choices and feel confident that you are optimising your health and well-being as you get back in shape and follow a sensible postnatal fitness program that's right for you.

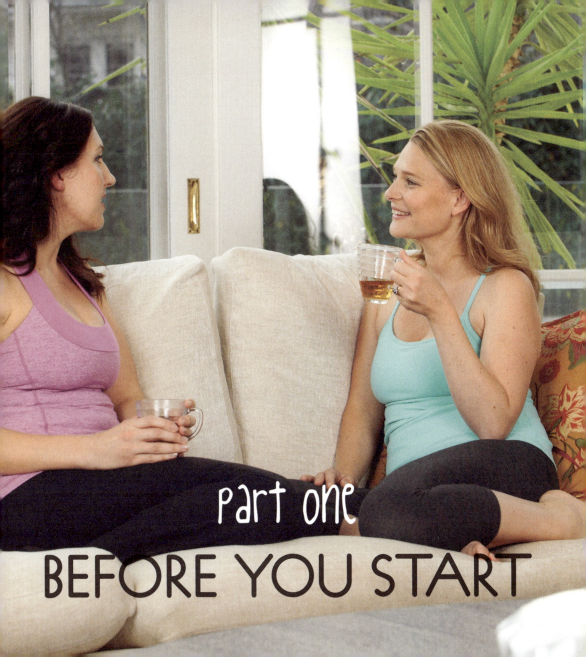

part one
BEFORE YOU START

Pregnancy, labour and delivery

Your pregnancy

If you were able to follow a sensible exercise plan during your pregnancy you will have reaped the benefits of staying active and be in a good position for getting back in shape now. If you were unable to exercise during pregnancy or you had to modify your activity levels you will need to start even more gently and build up gradually.

Regardless of prior activity, certain changes, such as lengthening and weakening of your abdominals and pelvic floor, affect all pregnant women and must be considered before jumping back into action.

You will also need to continue to accommodate any unresolved prenatal conditions, such as pelvic-joint pain or abdominal separation.

Labour of love

Labour is a demanding physical and emotional event. Had you just run a marathon, you would give yourself several days to rest and recover. Labour is no different – your body has endured a long and tiring workout, your mind has had to stay focused on the job at hand and you may have sustained a degree of soft-tissue damage and inflammation.

Labours vary significantly in their style, intensity and length. It stands to reason that a longer labour will have been more tiring and so require more rest and recovery. A longer second 'pushing' stage puts extra stress on your pelvic floor – while all postnatal women need to prioritise their pelvic-floor recovery, those who had to push for longer will need to give this vital muscle group even more care and attention.

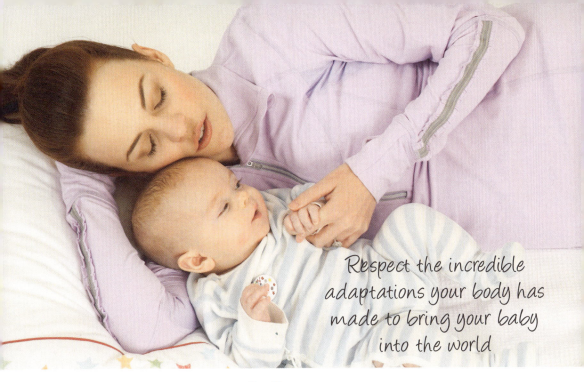

Respect the incredible adaptations your body has made to bring your baby into the world

Delivery

A range of circumstances may have necessitated intervention – epidural, episiotomy, forceps, caesarean – to help bring your baby into the world. It is helpful to remember that while your baby's birth may not have gone as you planned it will have been what was best for both of your well-being. Needless to say, longer time frames and extra care are in order after a delivery that required extra assistance. Even after a straightforward vaginal delivery you will almost certainly have a degree of perineal bruising and swelling, so although different deliveries require different recovery times and postnatal care, prioritising healing and deep-muscle recovery before fitness and toning is the rule for all.

Looking after yourself, as well as your baby

Looking after your new baby can be all-consuming. While you are establishing feeding routines and juggling sleep with the needs of your bub and the rest of the family, it is easy to put yourself last. To look after others, you must first nurture your own physical and emotional well-being.

Sleep, rest, exercise and good nutrition are all linked; when you are tired you are more likely to reach for the wrong food, when you exercise you sleep better and feel more energised, when you eat well you feel more like exercising and so on. Realistic expectations, time for yourself, a healthy diet and plenty of rest all complement safe sensible exercise.

Looking after yourself is the best gift you can give yourself, your baby and your family

Realistic goals and time frames

Many new mums are eager to lose weight and return to their pre-pregnancy fitness, body shape and activity levels, but too much, too soon can hinder rather than help your recovery. Pushing your body too much before it is ready can lead to short- and long-term physical problems such as incontinence and back pain. Expecting too much of yourself can leave you feeling sad, stressed and disappointed.

Realistic goals and exercise plans, based on understanding and listening to your body, will optimise the quality and speed of your recovery. Take the time to settle into motherhood and breastfeeding, allow yourself to enjoy these precious weeks and months and be gentle on your soul.

Sensible exercise after having a baby, using realistic goals and time frames, has many benefits, but you need to be patient with your body. It has been changing for nine months, so why not allow nine months to recover?

Be patient and listen to your body

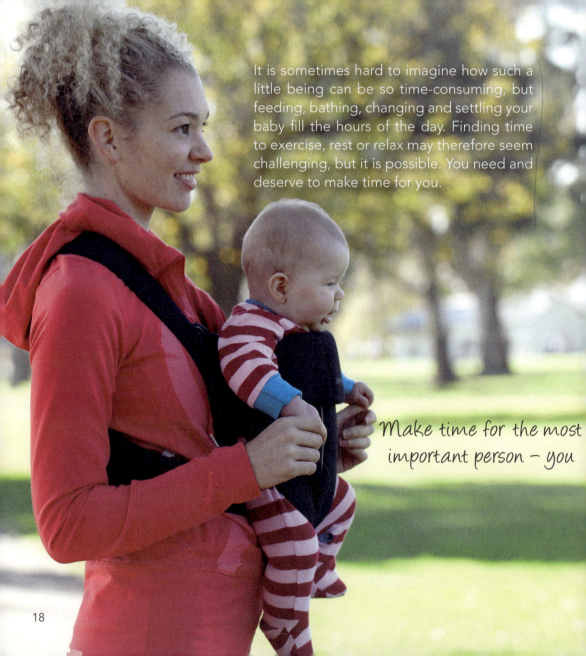

It is sometimes hard to imagine how such a little being can be so time-consuming, but feeding, bathing, changing and settling your baby fill the hours of the day. Finding time to exercise, rest or relax may therefore seem challenging, but it is possible. You need and deserve to make time for you.

Make time for the most important person – you

Tips for a happy, healthy you

The gift of time Family and friends want to help – so take them up on their offers to mind your baby, even for just half an hour, to allow you to rejuvenate with some rest, exercise, sleep or fresh air.

Sharing the caring Join a new-mums group. As well as regular get-togethers, take turns in looking after each other's babies to give you some time to yourself when someone else is looking after yours. On other days you can enjoy a walk in the park together.

Seize the moment Breaking up your exercise into short sessions – taking 10 minutes here and there – might be easier to fit into your day and gentler on your body. Listen to your body and use the time wisely. When your baby is sleeping, for example, should you do a few simple exercises or take a nap yourself?

Mum-and-bub fitness Exercising with your baby is a beautiful way to interact with each other while getting some fitness under your belt (pages 151-167).

Build exercise into your day Head out for a pram walk after a morning feed and later in the day perform a few simple strengthening exercises when your baby sleeps. Do pelvic-floor strengthening exercises while you're feeding and consciously check your posture and engage your core abdominals every time you change a nappy.

Group support Joining a mother-and-baby fitness class is a great way to enjoy appropriate exercise and meet some like-minded women.

Fatigue, sleep and energy levels

When you consider recovery from labour, broken sleep patterns, new responsibilities and breastfeeding, it is no surprise that new mums feel tired.

Performing a sensible level and quantity of exercise will boost your energy levels and improve your quality of sleep, whereas overdoing it may lead to exhaustion. Listen to your needs and find a healthy balance of rest, sleep and exercise. Avoid the temptation to 'keep on going'.

Tips to keep you feeling fresh

- Aim to get a little exercise and fresh air most days.
- Listen to your body and balance exercise and rest.
- Accept offers of help.
- Ask visitors to make their own cup of tea and bring yours to you on the couch.
- Work out which household chores really need doing and which ones can wait.
- Sleep if you can, rest if you can't.
- Practise relaxation – simple techniques can become a powerful tonic (page 168).

*Monitor how you're feeling
Be true to your needs – your body
and your baby will thank you*

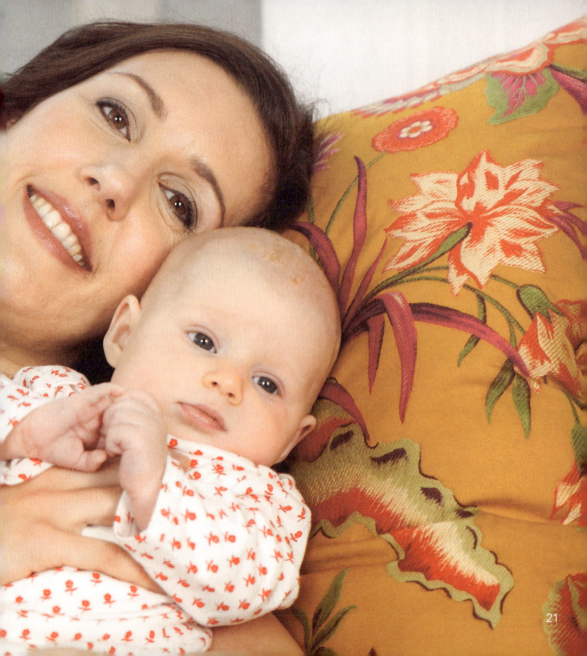

Mood and morale

Hormonal changes, fatigue and powerful emotions can play havoc with your mood. Feeling weepy or sad may be the last thing you expected after the joy and elation of your baby's arrival but it is not unusual to have 'the baby blues', days where you feel low and emotionally overwhelmed.

Usually a little TLC, a good cry, some fresh air and a few quiet days will leave you feeling happier and refreshed.

If you are feeling constantly sad or low, struggling to look after yourself or your baby, or you have any concerns about your mood, then talking to your partner, a friend or family member is helpful, but it is also important you seek assessment, advice and guidance from your doctor. There is no need to struggle on alone if you are experiencing postnatal depression.

Mood-lifting tips

- Appropriate exercise, time out and fresh air are all fabulous ways to boost your mood.
- Balance sleep, rest and activity.
- Recruit help and delegate responsibilities with household duties.
- Try some simple relaxation techniques.
- Remember that it's okay to cry.
- Talk to a friend.
- Meet with other mums.
- Seek advice if you are worried about your mood, health or your ability to look after yourself or your baby.
- Be gentle and kind to yourself – you are doing an amazing job.

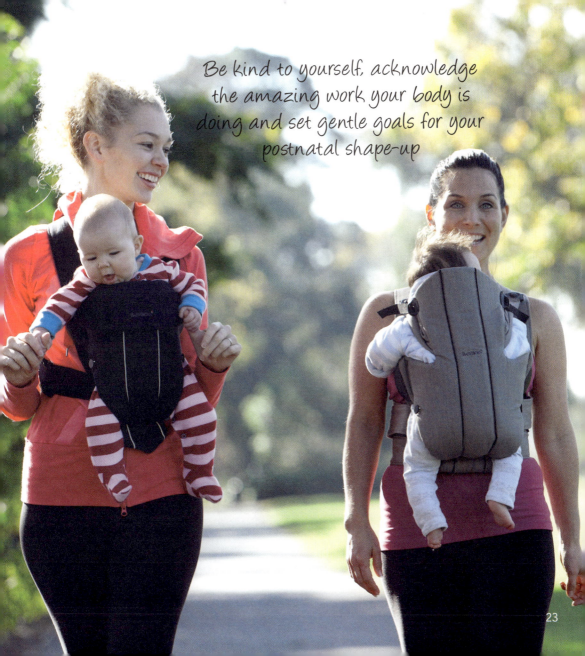
Be kind to yourself, acknowledge the amazing work your body is doing and set gentle goals for your postnatal shape-up

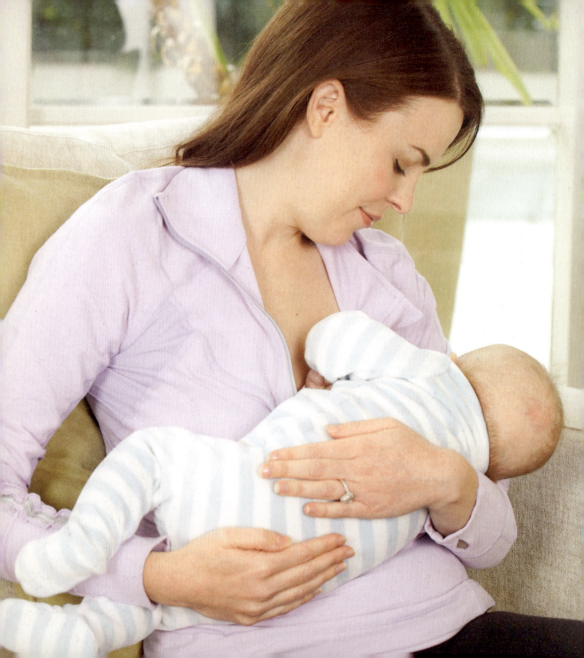

Breastfeeding

Feeding, by breast or bottle, is a wonderful time to relax and connect with your baby.

It is important to monitor your posture while feeding – poor positioning will take its toll. Avoid aches and pains by ensuring you are well-supported, allowing you to relax your neck and shoulders. You may use a small footstool, so that your knees are slightly higher than your hips, and a pillow under the arm that is supporting your baby. If you prefer lying down to feed, still aim for comfortable and well-supported body alignment.

Breastfeeding tips

- Stay well-hydrated – always drink a glass of water at each feed in addition to your usual intake and have an extra glass within reach.
- Check for good feeding posture – keep your spine long and your neck and shoulders relaxed.
- Sneak in a few pelvic-floor or core-abdominal exercises while feeding.
- Always wear a supportive underwire-free bra (as underwire may interfere with your milk ducts), especially if exercising.
- If you have a fever, or your breasts feel hot or uncomfortable, refrain from exercise and seek advice from your doctor immediately.
- Where possible, feed before exercise. It will help your baby to settle and you will feel more comfortable.

Nutrition and hydration

You will need plenty of energy over the coming months. A healthy, well-balanced diet and good hydration will complement your rest and exercise plan.

Whether you breast- or bottle-feed, a healthy diet of fresh fruit, vegetables, whole grains and lean protein will help you recover and meet the energy demands you need to look after and enjoy your baby. Include a range of nutritious foods and check with your doctor if you think you require vitamins or supplements. (If you are breastfeeding you need to add approximately 300 calories – e.g. one tuna-and-salad sandwich – a day, on top of your pre-pregnancy requirements.)

Hydration is important for all mums. If you are breastfeeding, drink a glass of water at each breastfeed in addition to your regular intake.

You may be keen to lose a few extra pregnancy kilos but now is no time for crash diets. While some mums seem to magically drop weight while breastfeeding, and others after they have finished breastfeeding, this is not the case for everyone. There is no rush. Be patient – a healthy diet, sensible activity and realistic time frames matter most.

Celebrate your body's changes and what it has achieved – you will get back in shape, in good time.

Enjoy a healthy, well-balanced diet and drink plenty of H_2O

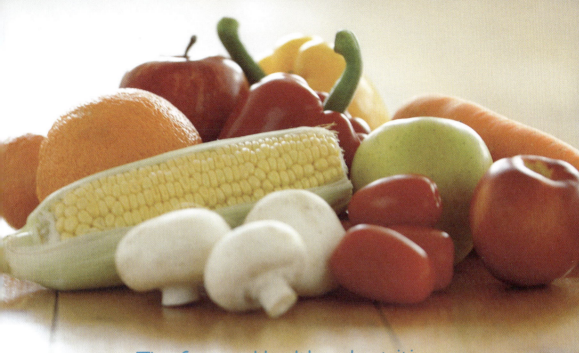

Tips for good health and nutrition

- Drink plenty of fresh water – try adding a sprig of mint or slice of lemon.
- Keep your water bottle by your side.
- Avoid long periods without eating.
- Sleep, rest and frequent healthy snacks will help you stay energised and avoid the blood-sugar drops that tempt you to reach for the wrong food.
- Stock up with plenty of user-friendly, fresh options in your fridge and pantry.
- Get out into the fresh air – it's a tonic for your soul.

Extra-special thought

Certain muscle groups and postnatal conditions deserve extra consideration and attention in your post-baby shape-up plan.

Your fitness overhaul starts on the inside. Regaining the strength and function of your pelvic floor and core-stabilising muscles is your highest priority. These muscles are the foundation support for all activity and exercise. Working outer muscles before you have regained inner strength and control can lead to injury and incontinence. It is also important that you attend to any new or ongoing musculoskeletal aches and pains, and that your exercise program aids rather than hinders their rehabilitation.

Foundations first – accommodate accordingly

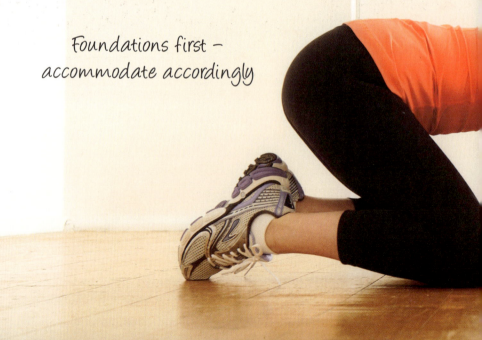

Pelvic floor first

The pelvic floor is a muscular sling that supports the bladder, bowel and uterus. Its integrity and strength is vital for continence (bladder and bowel control), core stability and sexual function. The pelvic-floor muscles are lengthened and weakened during pregnancy and childbirth – one in three mothers suffers incontinence as a result. Even if you had a caesarean section your pelvic floor will have been stretched under the load of your growing baby for nine months, so it is essential that every new mum puts her pelvic floor first.

Immediately after having your baby your pelvic floor is compromised, placing you at increased risk of not only incontinence, but also prolapse and back pain. This will be more so if you had a long second (pushing) stage during labour, a difficult delivery, a large baby or if this is not your first child. The good news is there's plenty you can do to regain healthy pelvic-floor strength and function.

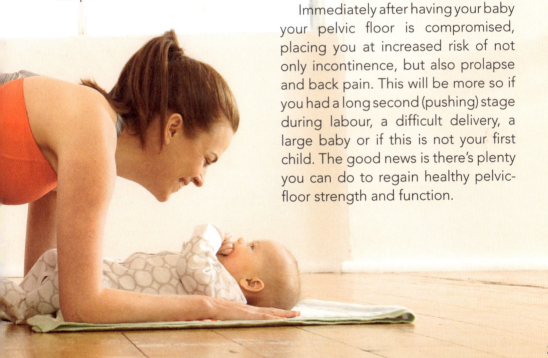

Exercise and your pelvic floor

Exercise can help or hinder

While it's tempting to quickly return to energetic high-impact exercise and strength training, nothing could be worse for your pelvic floor. Even if you have no leakage or embarrassing moments now, doing too much too soon predisposes you to incontinence later. Take your time and be patient. You must regain pelvic-floor strength and control first.

A sensible fitness plan and time frame prioritises pelvic-floor recovery. Your pelvic floor plays a significant role in exercise and daily life – it must be strong enough to resist the downward pressure created by activities such as running, lifting and coughing. With correct retraining, in time you will be able to return to all exercise. As a guide, you can resume an activity if you are able to maintain a pelvic-floor contraction (lift) throughout the action. For some moves, such as running or abdominal curls, this won't be until after eight to 12 weeks or more. Don't worry – there are plenty of other fitness activities you can do in the meantime.

Try to perform pelvic-floor strengthening exercises daily, return to exercise sensibly and gradually and avoid any action that weakens these muscles.

Short-term patience for long-term control

Exercises and activities to avoid while your pelvic floor recovers

Certain exercises place significant stress on your pelvic floor and should be avoided until it has completely recovered. (This may take several months.)
- Bouncy high-impact moves such as running, jumping and energetic aerobics.
- Lifting anything heavier than your baby.
- Straining on the toilet.
- Straining or holding your breath while you exercise.
- Abdominal curls.
- Lunges and wide squats.
- Heavy strength-training.
- Chronic coughing.

Pelvic-floor fitness tips

Rest up Avoid standing for long periods of time and put your feet up whenever you get the chance.

In the bathroom Straining due to constipation can lead to pelvic-floor weakness or even prolapse. Take your time on the toilet. Drinking plenty of water, having a high-fibre diet and sensible exercise will help.

Heavy lifting Avoid lifting anything heavier than your baby for three months. Find creative ways to lighten the load – carry your baby in a sling instead of a (heavier) capsule, use more shopping bags with less in each, ask for help.

Work out without bounce High-impact moves such as running, energetic aerobics and jumping are disastrous for a vulnerable pelvic floor. Refrain from such exercise until you pass the 'pelvic-floor ready' test (page 127). Instead, as your fitness improves, increase your training intensity by adding swimming and power walking or incorporating hills or stairs into your daily walk. Your breasts will thank you too.

Strain, no gain Exercises that increase intra-abdominal pressure will further compromise a weak pelvic floor. Make sure you are not pushing down on your pelvic floor, nor holding your breath.

Pelvic-floor strengthening — make it part of your day If you do nothing else, be sure you exercise your pelvic floor daily.

The knack In the early postnatal days you may find your pelvic floor needs a little extra support, so place your hand on the outside of your clothing to support stressful actions such as sneezing or coughing.

Check it out In the early days after delivery, ask your midwife or doctor to check your perineum and visually assess whether or not you are lifting your pelvic floor. Arrange to see a women's health physiotherapist as soon as possible if you are unsure about pelvic-floor exercise technique or have any concerns at all. At your six weeks' medical follow-up you will benefit from an internal check of your pelvic-floor strength.

Gradual progression Gradually progress your exercises according to your pelvic-floor control, only adding a movement if you are able to lift your pelvic floor and maintain the lift throughout the entire action.

Technique matters It is very important not only that you do pelvic-floor exercises three times per day, but also that you do them correctly (page 66).

The ins and outs of abdominals

Recovery from the inside out

You are not alone if you are keen to get your waist back and your tummy flat but after nine months of stretching your abdominal muscles need time to return to their pre-pregnancy state.

The abdominal muscles are arranged in four layers. The outer layers – the rectus abdominus and external obliques – are the ones you can see and are responsible for bending and twisting movements such as sit-ups. The innermost layer – the transverse abdominus – works with deep back muscles and the pelvic floor to stabilise and support your spine. The internal obliques are the second-deepest abdominal group and play a role in both movement and stability. Deep-abdominal rehabilitation must occur before you work your outer abdominals.

The stretching of your abdominals during pregnancy leaves them weakened after delivery, so although you might be tempted to do sit-ups and crunches straight after having your baby it would be detrimental to your recovery. Not only would it put stress on your pelvic floor, it would also compromise your core stability, thus slowing your all-important deep-muscle recovery and making you more vulnerable to back pain, incontinence and prolapse.

These muscles will need even longer if you had a particularly large baby, twins or a caesarean delivery, if you have back pain or an abdominal separation, or if your abdominal muscles did not recover fully after a prior pregnancy (page 36).

As your foundation strength improves you can gradually add outer-muscle training (e.g. a biceps curl) while engaging and sustaining core recruitment, but it is at least eight to 12 weeks before most women have the underlying pelvic-floor and core strength to support abdominal curls and other exercises that load the spine and increase intra-abdominal pressure. This will be even longer if you have had a caesarean section or an abdominal separation. You should have worked through the core exercises on pages 74 to 81 before attempting outer-abdominal training.

Engage Your Core

Foundations first

Your deepest abdominal layer is responsible for spinal stability. It works with your deep back muscles and pelvic floor to function as a low, muscular corset that supports your spine and pelvis. After the stretching and weakening of pregnancy these deep muscles will struggle to sustain the spinal support that is required during mainstream exercises. Rehabilitation of these muscles with low-load exercises is therefore vital. Focusing on your core and pelvic floor before anything else is like building strong foundations before you build your house.

Quality not quantity

Correct core-muscle recruitment involves a gentle in-drawing of the deep muscles around your lower abdomen, with a simultaneous pelvic-floor lift. It is felt internally between your naval and your pubic bone but no outer activity should be seen. The stronger action of sucking in your ribs and waist uses outer abdominals and will not assist your core-strength recovery.

Start with simple core recruitment (page 72). Soon you will be able to switch on your core in several positions and gradually increase the challenge. Only progress when you have excellent quality and control. If you notice any signs of loss of form, go back to the previous level. Your eventual aim is to be able to recruit your core and maintain it during all activities and exercises.

Tips for core training

- Breathe normally.
- Maintain a long spine and natural lumbar curve.
- Avoid unwanted muscle activity such as shoulder shrugging, sucking in your rib cage or clenching your gluteals/buttocks.
- Check for good posture.
- Keep all movement smooth and controlled.

As well as exercising your core formally, build its training into your day, drawing your lower abdomen gently inwards every time you walk through a door or feed your baby.

Abdominal muscle separation

Your abdominals are united along their midline by a strong fibrous sheath, the linea alba, which becomes thinner as it stretches during pregnancy. It is not unusual for a separation, or gap, to develop, most commonly above or below the navel, known as a rectus abdominus diastasis.

Over half of new mothers have a separation in the first few days after birth, but many resolve quickly as the uterus reduces in size, so that only 36 per cent still have this at six weeks. Women with a diastasis have even less underlying muscle strength, further compromising abdominal-wall function and spinal stability. This means they are more vulnerable to poor posture, spinal and pelvic instability, back pain and injury. If this applies to you, then spinal stabilisation and recovery of the separation must be your focus; overloading the outer abdominals with inappropriate exercises such as abdominal curls can hinder resolution and increase the diastasis.

To test for a diastasis:

- Lie on your back with your feet on the floor, knees slightly bent.
- Place your fingers along the midline of your abdomen.
- Slowly lift your head and shoulders, feeling for a gap or bulge above or below your naval.
- Turn your fingers to run across the separation to measure the gap in finger widths.
- A space two fingers wide or more is considered significant and requires extra exercise modification.
- Your physiotherapist may recommend wearing a support garment.

Exercise and abdominal separation

Engage your deep abdominals and pelvic floor during all daily activities, especially lifting.

Start with core stability training in static positions (page 74) then gradually add gentle challenges such as an arm raise in four-point kneeling or leg raise while sitting on a fitball.

Check with your women's health physiotherapist before you progress your exercise program.

Emphasise quality control – if you lose your deep-abdominal recruitment, find yourself holding your breath, losing form or using unwanted muscles or your diastasis is increasing or bulging then take it back a level.

Avoid all exercises that work your outer abdominals or load your back. Exercises such as abdominal curls, obliques curls, hovers and push-ups should not be resumed until:

- your diastasis is less than two finger widths;
- you are free of back pain;
- you have regained strong core control;
- you are able to sustain sound core recruitment throughout the exercise;
- the separation does not increase or bulge when you perform the move.

Posture and back health

While a pregnant woman is more likely to experience lower-back pain, it is your upper back that is vulnerable now. The activities of a new mum – leaning forward over the change table, floor or bath and feeding your baby, for example – play havoc with your back, neck and shoulders. Also, pregnancy hormones continue to soften your ligaments and increase joint laxity, making you more at risk of aches and injury.

Look after your back

Monitor your posture. Always lengthen your spine and roll your shoulders gently back and down.

- Stand or sit tall, especially when you are feeding.
- Stretch to correct poor posture frequently.
- Perform stretches such as the chest stretch (page 172) to combat the leaning-forward lifestyle of a new mum.
- Avoid slouching by visualising a long spine and lifting your chest.
- Engage your core and pelvic floor whenever you think of it, especially when you are lifting or exercising.
- Lift nothing heavier than your baby for at least six weeks.
- Get help with heavy loads and take extra care to check your posture and engage your core when you are lifting the pram, carrying your baby and so on.

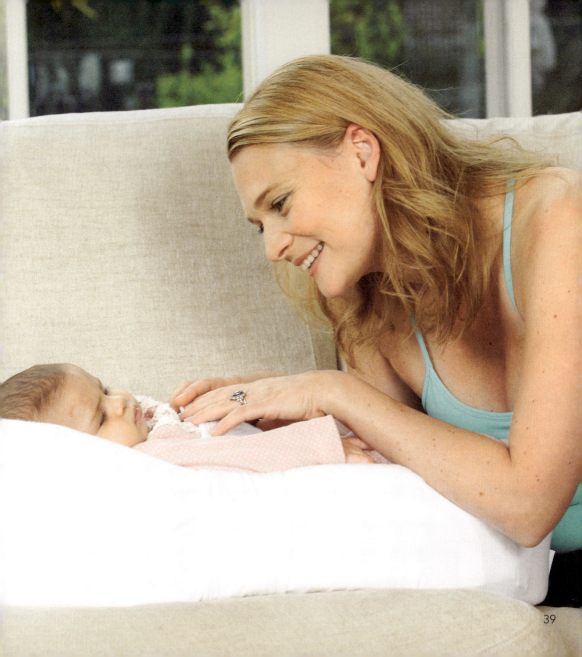

Looking after your pelvic joints

Some women experience pain and a feeling of instability in their pelvic joints during pregnancy or labour. This is due to a number of contributing factors: pregnancy hormones that cause joint laxity, extra load on the joints as your baby grows plus compromised muscular support and stability. Pregnancy-related pelvic-joint pain can range in intensity. Unfortunately this does not necessarily resolve spontaneously after delivery but sensible exercise can help recovery.

Avoid exercises that cause or aggravate pelvic-joint pain, including standing for periods of time, walking, going up and down steps, wide-based activities such as wide squats or lunges, asymmetrical or single-leg weight-bearing exercises and any activities that tend to rotate the pelvis.

Helpful hints

- Select narrow-based exercises (feet no wider than hip-width apart).
- Avoid standing or kneeling on one leg – choose options that bear weight evenly between left and right.
- Focus on your core and pelvic floor as these muscles help pelvic stability.
- Work on the fitball or in the water. They are less stressful and involve extra stability training.
- See your physiotherapist if you are in any doubt about which exercises are right for you.

Other concerns

Ensure that any discomfort or concern you have is assessed by your health-care provider and check that the exercise you do is helping not exacerbating an existing condition.

De Quervain's tenosynovitis is an inflammatory, over-use condition involving the tendons of the thumb, near the wrist. It is thought to occur more in new mothers due to lifting, carrying and supporting their baby, but several other activities may aggravate or cause it, such as turning keys and door knobs, opening jars and knitting. Try to avoid, or take frequent breaks from, aggravating activities. Icing the area 15 minutes twice per day, practising self-massage and forearm stretches, as guided by your physiotherapist, will help.

Carpal tunnel syndrome is another condition that can affect the hand and forearm in pre- and postnatal women. Compression of the nerves and blood vessels that supply your hand may lead to pain, altered sensation and weakness.

With either condition you should avoid using hand weights and find alternatives to exercises that involve weight-bearing through your hand or wrist. A wrist brace or medication may also be recommended to assist comfort for daily activities.

Postnatal Exercise Guidelines

While you might like a specific date for when you will be ready to return to various activities, everyone is different (depending on your pregnancy, labour, recovery, energy levels, the baby's health and more). This book therefore aims to help you understand your individual needs and their exercise implications so you can make wise choices about getting back in shape within the time frames that are right for you.

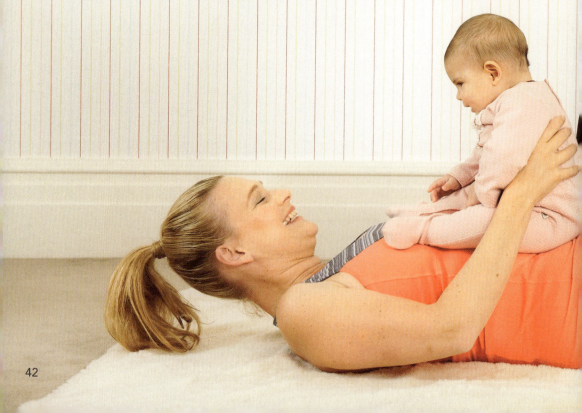

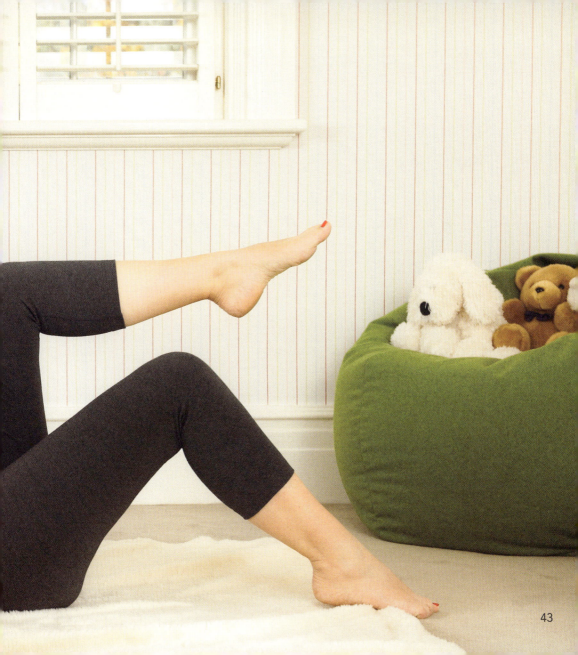

The early days

The early days after delivery are a time for rest and recovery. It is vital that you allow soft tissue to heal and your energy levels to recover before resuming exercise. The main areas for care are your pelvic floor and perineum, which may be bruised and swollen. At the same time your breasts will be changing as your milk comes in and your baby learns to suckle. So for at least two days (longer if you had a difficult delivery or a caesarean section) lie back, rest up and allow your body to heal and recover.

If you have suffered any soft-tissue inflammation in the perineal area apply the RICER principle, just as you would any soft-tissue injury after sport:

R   Rest
I   Ice – small ice packs/frozen, water-filled condoms wrapped in soft material, placed against your perineum will help decrease swelling, discomfort and bruising
C   Compression also helps decrease swelling and bruising – comfortable but firm underpants can provide effective compression to the perineal area
E   Elevation – to help decrease swelling and pain, be horizontal as much as possible, with your feet up
R   Referral – if you have any aches, pains or concerns post-delivery seek assessment and advice from your doctor, physiotherapist or midwife

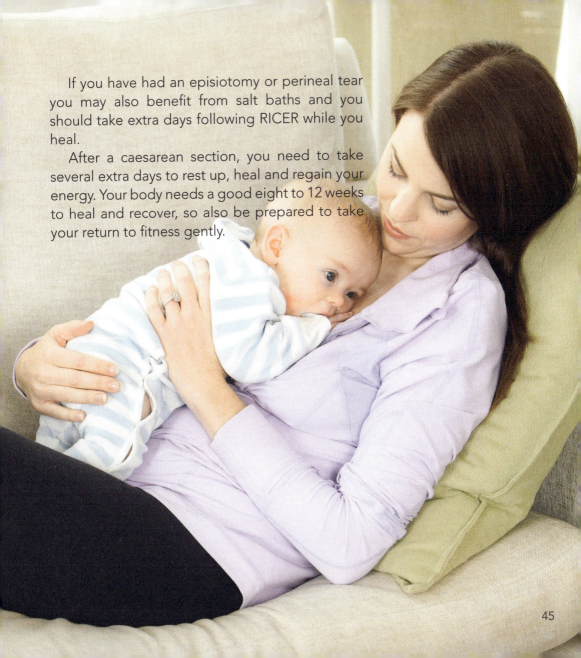

If you have had an episiotomy or perineal tear you may also benefit from salt baths and you should take extra days following RICER while you heal.

After a caesarean section, you need to take several extra days to rest up, heal and regain your energy. Your body needs a good eight to 12 weeks to heal and recover, so also be prepared to take your return to fitness gently.

Early weeks

In the first few weeks, focus on pelvic-floor and core strengthening. Your baby and settling in may keep you active enough but you can add mobility exercises and light daily walks when you feel fine.

It is important to avoid straining your back, pelvic floor and body in general. One guideline is to lift nothing heavier than your baby for a good six weeks or longer and not to perform any activity until your deep abdominals and pelvic floor can stay switched on throughout.

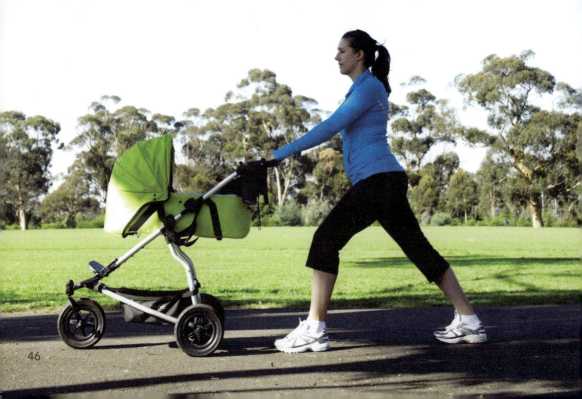

As the weeks turn to months

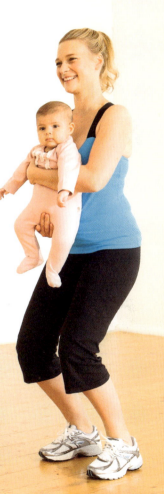

As you become stronger you will be able to build on your fitness slowly, gradually adding a variety of sensible exercises. After six weeks or so, you can progress as your body dictates; varying your core exercises, adding more walking and other cardiovascular fitness styles and beginning light strengthening options and stretches. From here on you will gradually build more exercises into your routine. Everyone is unique, so rather than time lines, this book provides guidelines that will allow you to understand and recognise when you are ready to progress.

After eight to 12 weeks you should be able to enjoy a fitness routine three to four times per week, which incorporates a variety of low-impact options and sensible strength training.

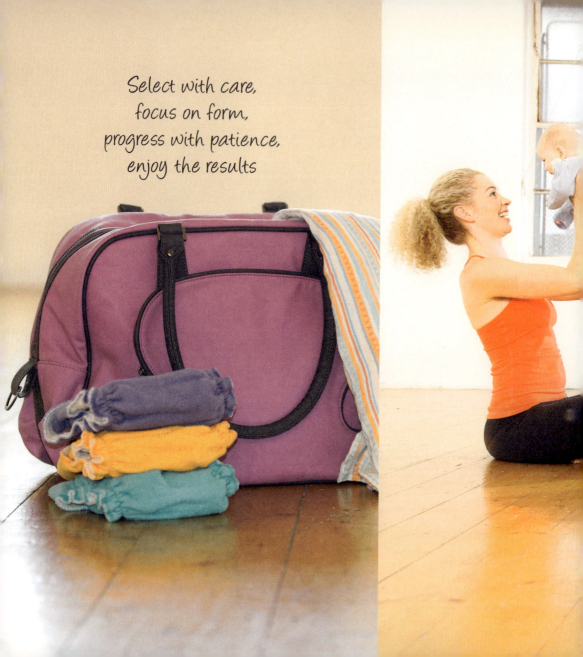

Select with care,
focus on form,
progress with patience,
enjoy the results

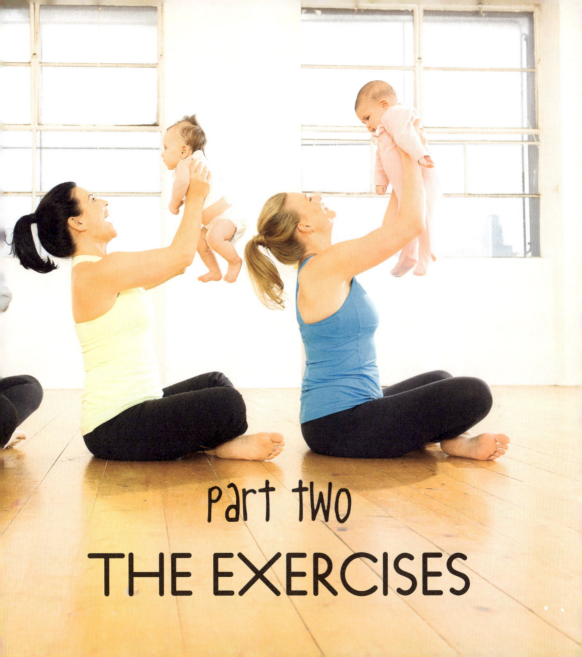

part two
THE EXERCISES

Optimise your recovery and return to fitness

The following section includes a range of exercises to match your postnatal situation, fitness level and goals. Alongside the important pelvic floor, core stability and specific strength exercises, you will find a comprehensive range of mobility, cardiovascular, strengthening and flexibility options that will safely guide you towards feeling fitter and stronger. Relaxation tips are also included to help you make the most of your precious time out.

Equipment – such as fitballs, exercise bands and light dumb-bells – is used in some exercises, but there are also equipment-free alternatives.

Technique tips, modifications and progressions allow you to optimise your form and lighten or increase the challenge to suit your individual fitness and ability.

Stretching is an important element of fitness and should be performed after exercise. Appropriate stretches are suggested to complement certain exercises.

There are also hints for returning to the gym, fitness classes and the pool, plus specific guidelines as to when you can return to high-impact exercise, weights and abdominal curls.

There are two sections unique to this book: 'Working out with your baby' allows you to interact while you exercise, and 'Stroller fitness' helps to boost your fitness while you are out and about.

Exercise for the weakest link

Regardless of your outer-muscle strength you should not lift weights or perform exercises that compromise a weak pelvic floor or an abdominal seperation. The rule of thumb is to accommodate for the weakest link, always choosing exercises that don't put pressure on that area.

Remember you are unique – your health, fitness and energy levels will be different to the next person's. You must allow your body to heal and get strong, one step at a time.

Be true to your body and be kind to your soul

> Keep your doctor informed about your exercise program and seek professional advice if you have any discomfort or concern. If you are unsure about your exercise selection or technique check it out with your physiotherapist.

Mobility

Enjoy these moves throughout your day

Gentle mobility exercises can be used to prevent or relieve joint stiffness and muscle tightness. They also serve as a light exercise option in the early days after delivery or when you need to take it easy. Moving your joints through their full range of motion helps to keep them supple. Later, when your fitness has progressed, such exercises will be an effective way to warm up and cool down as a complement to other more strenuous exercises.

Focus on slow, flowing movement when following each of these mobility exercises.

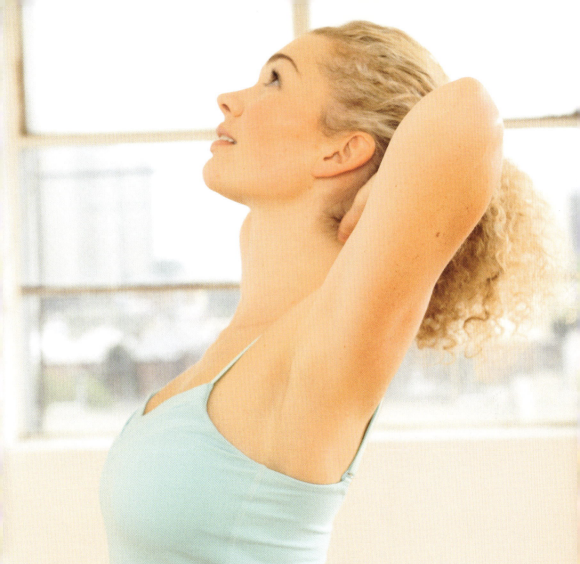
Ease away the tension

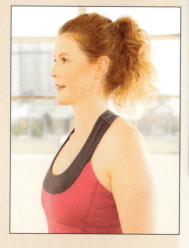

Shoulder rolls

Starting position
- Sitting or standing tall, elongate your spine.

Action
- Roll your shoulders slowly up, back and down.
- 10 repetitions.

Neck stretch

Starting position
- Sit or stand tall.

Action
- Looking straight ahead, tilt your head sideways taking your ear towards your shoulder.
- To improve the stretch, push your opposite arm and shoulder downwards as though you are holding a heavy suitcase.
- Hold for 5 slow breaths then stretch to the other side.
- 3 repetitions each way.

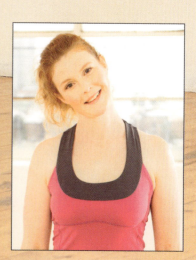

Climb the ladder

Starting position
- Sit or stand tall.
- Bend your elbows by your sides, pointing hands upwards.

Action
- Draw your shoulder blades down (the opposite of shrugging).
- Reach one arm upwards as you pull your opposite elbow down and in towards your hip.
- Gently stretch your body side to side, slowly reaching one arm then the other, as though climbing a ladder.

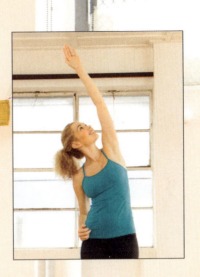

Wake-up stretch

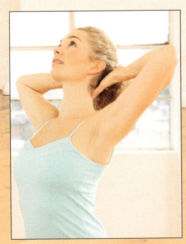

Starting position
- Sit or stand tall and place your fingers behind your ears.

Action
- Elongate your spine, draw your elbows backwards.
- Gently arch your upper back and look upwards, supporting your head with your hands.
- Hold for 5 slow breaths then relax.
- 3 repetitions.

Upper-back rotation

Starting position
- Sit or stand tall and place your fingers behind your ears.

Action
- Elongate your spine, draw your elbows backwards and shoulder blades downwards.
- Draw your lower abdomen towards your lower back to engage your core.
- Rotate your upper back as far as is comfortable to look behind you.
- Slowly rotate your upper back side to side, keeping your lower back and pelvis stable.
- Turn to each side 5 times.

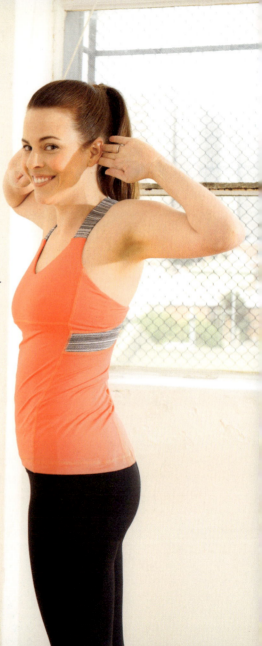

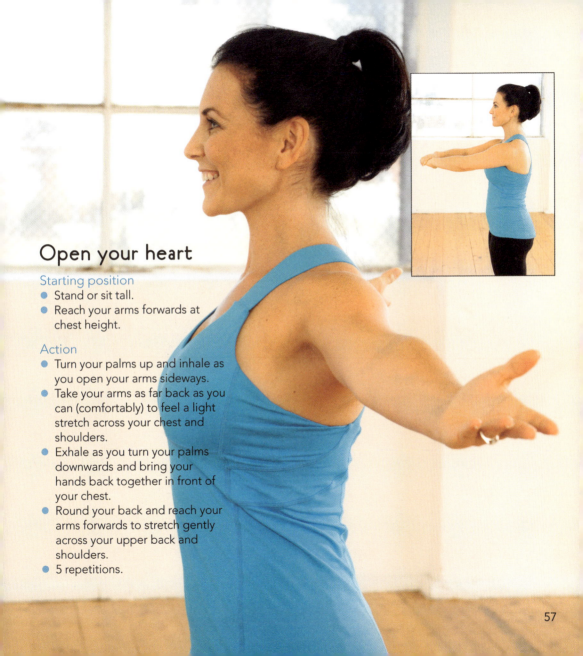

Open your heart

Starting position
- Stand or sit tall.
- Reach your arms forwards at chest height.

Action
- Turn your palms up and inhale as you open your arms sideways.
- Take your arms as far back as you can (comfortably) to feel a light stretch across your chest and shoulders.
- Exhale as you turn your palms downwards and bring your hands back together in front of your chest.
- Round your back and reach your arms forwards to stretch gently across your upper back and shoulders.
- 5 repetitions.

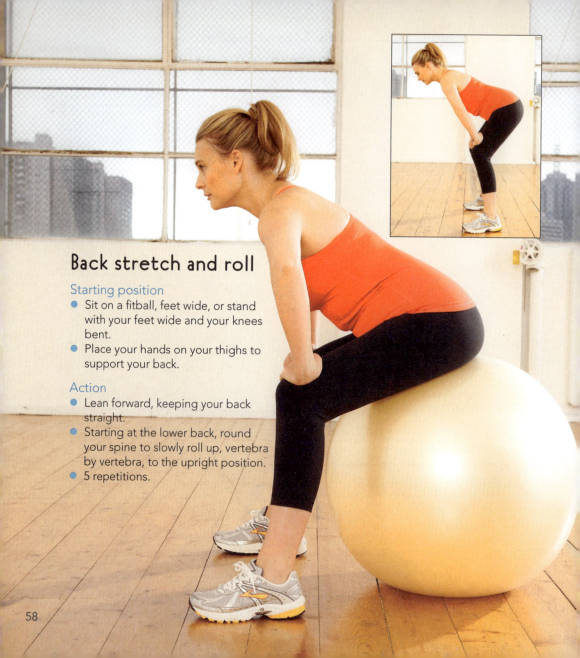

Back stretch and roll

Starting position
- Sit on a fitball, feet wide, or stand with your feet wide and your knees bent.
- Place your hands on your thighs to support your back.

Action
- Lean forward, keeping your back straight.
- Starting at the lower back, round your spine to slowly roll up, vertebra by vertebra, to the upright position.
- 5 repetitions.

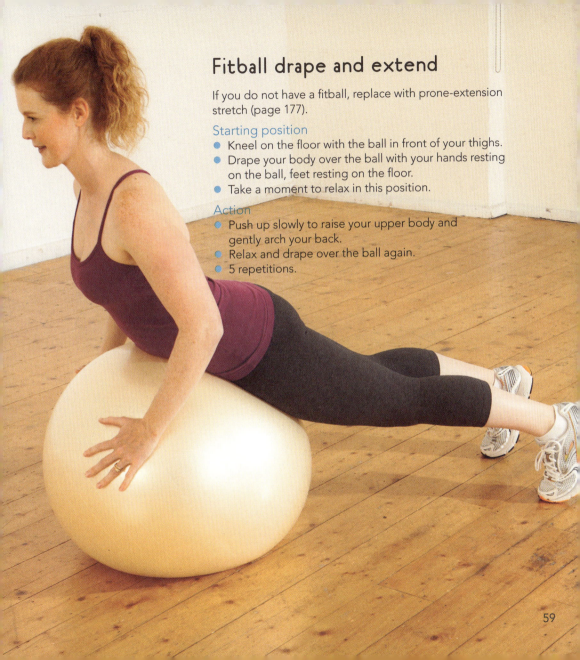

Fitball drape and extend

If you do not have a fitball, replace with prone-extension stretch (page 177).

Starting position
- Kneel on the floor with the ball in front of your thighs.
- Drape your body over the ball with your hands resting on the ball, feet resting on the floor.
- Take a moment to relax in this position.

Action
- Push up slowly to raise your upper body and gently arch your back.
- Relax and drape over the ball again.
- 5 repetitions.

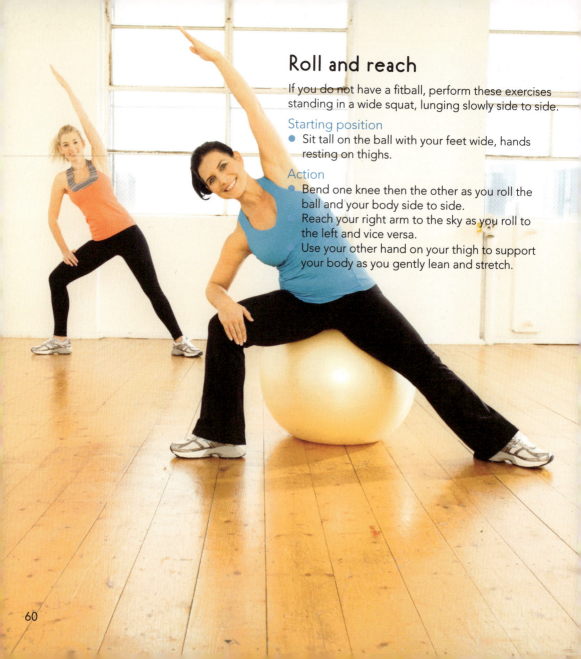

Roll and reach

If you do not have a fitball, perform these exercises standing in a wide squat, lunging slowly side to side.

Starting position
- Sit tall on the ball with your feet wide, hands resting on thighs.

Action
- Bend one knee then the other as you roll the ball and your body side to side.
- Reach your right arm to the sky as you roll to the left and vice versa.
- Use your other hand on your thigh to support your body as you gently lean and stretch.

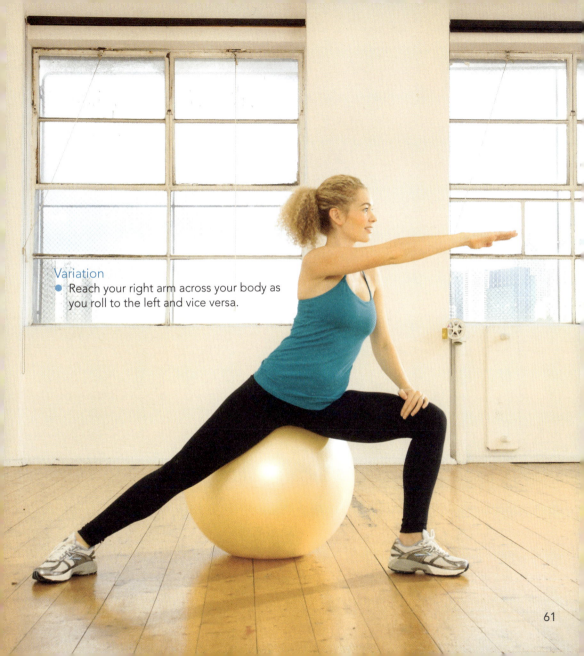

Variation
- Reach your right arm across your body as you roll to the left and vice versa.

Posture, core and pelvic floor

The foundations of healthy movement and control

Your deep abdominals and pelvic floor are the foundations of movement and function. They are responsible for supporting your spine as well as bladder and bowel control, working together to prevent back pain, injury and incontinence. Therefore your first step towards regaining your prenatal fitness and body shape must be to regain their strength and function. As your fitness and strength improve, your core and pelvic-floor exercises can also progress so that eventually you will be able to hold a stronger pelvic-floor lift for longer and perform more challenging core exercises.

Never perform an exercise unless you are able to engage and maintain pelvic-floor and deep-abdominal recruitment throughout.

Having good posture is also imperative for an ache- and injury-free return to fitness and daily activities. Checking and correcting your posture, whether you are at rest or exercising, will help you stay comfortable and optimise your health and fitness regime.

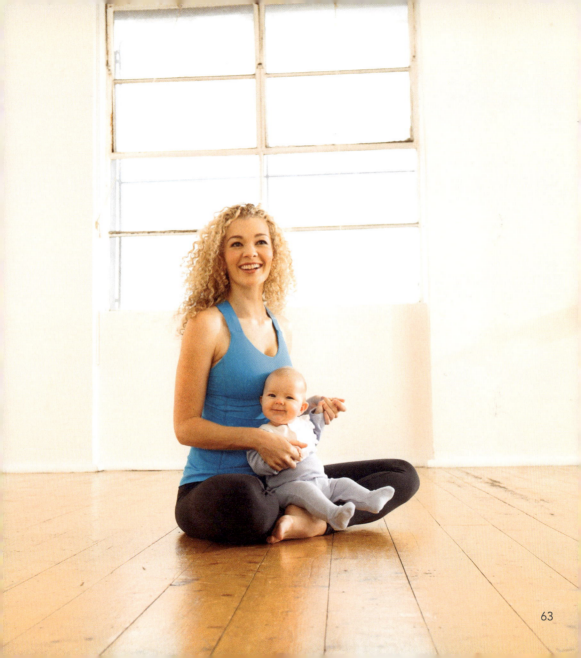

Posture perfect

Posture and movement awareness are the key to staying injury-free and being able to move easily with fine form. New mums are particularly at risk of neck, shoulder and upper-back pain due to leaning forwards over their baby so often. Become attuned to how you are holding and moving your body and regularly run through the following posture body check.

Head and neck
- Keep your neck long and in line with your spine, and your shoulders relaxed, back and down.
- Avoid shrugging your shoulders, poking your chin forward or tilting your head downwards.

Back and pelvis
- Lengthen your spine.
- Avoid slouching or rounding your upper back – keep your chest up and stand tall.
- Check that your pelvis and lower back are in neutral alignment, with the natural lumbar curve present but not exaggerated.

When you are standing, check that your spine is long, the weight is spread evenly through your feet and your knees are soft (not locked straight).

Lengthen your spine, lift up your heart and relax your neck and shoulders

Lift up your heart

Starting position
- Stand with your feet hip-width apart.

Action
- Spread the weight evenly between your feet and toes.
- Soften your knees.
- Breathing normally, lightly in-draw your lower abdomen and lift your pelvic floor.
- Imagine a helium balloon attached to the top of your head, helping you to lengthen your spine, and raise your chest to 'lift up your heart'.
- Settle your shoulder blades gently back and down.
- Check your tail bone is slightly tucked under and your natural lumbar curve is present.
- Hold for 5 slow breaths.
- Check your posture in this way often, especially after leaning over your baby.

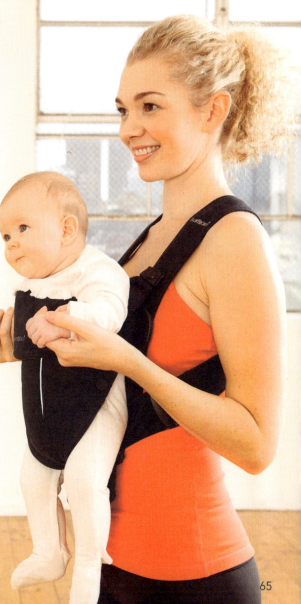

Pelvic floor

The pelvic floor is out of sight, but it must not be out of mind. You can help your pelvic floor regain strength and function by avoiding activities that stress the muscles and by performing effective pelvic-floor strengthening exercises every day. Correct technique is vital. Avoid the common mistake of pushing down instead of lifting as this will weaken rather than strengthen your pelvic floor. For best results see a women's health physiotherapist, who will give you individual advice and instruction to ensure you are optimising your return to a fit and healthy you, inside and out.

Pelvic-floor training tips

Technique
- You should feel a lifting and closing sensation, similar to when you are trying to control wind or hold on when you need to go to the toilet.
- Always check your spine is long and your lower back is in the neutral (natural lumbar curve) position.
- Breathe normally.
- These muscles are internal, so do not expect to see movement when you switch them on.
- Make each pelvic-floor contraction as strong as possible.
- Relax your pelvic floor completely between each lift and for at least as long as you hold the lift.
- Aim for quality not quantity.

Put your pelvic floor first

Avoid
- Straining or pushing down on your pelvic floor.
- Holding your breath.
- Squeezing your buttocks or inner-thigh muscles.
- Sucking in your ribs and waist.
- Tensing your neck or shoulders, hands, feet or any other muscles.

Visualise
- Lifting the muscular sling towards your heart.
- Drawing your tail bone and pubic bone inwards and upwards.
- Trying to stop the flow of urine or control wind.

Cross-train your pelvic floor – slow and fast
- Your pelvic floor needs strength for all-day control, plus the ability to provide fast, strong support when you cough, laugh or sneeze.
- Functional training involves incorporating both long holds and quick lifts into your daily routine.

Progress
As you feel able:
- Increase the strength of each lift.
- Increase the hold time of the long holds.
- Switch on the muscles faster for the quick lifts.
- Increase the number of repetitions per set.
- Try a new or more challenging position.
- Decrease the rest time between each lift (but always rest for at least as long as the hold time).

Exercise and daily life

- Always engage your core and pelvic floor when you cough, laugh, sneeze, bend down, lift or exercise.
- Refrain from the load or activity if you are unable to sustain a pelvic-floor contraction throughout.
- Incorporating pelvic-floor exercises into your daily activities is one way to make sure they happen – when you are feeding, waiting for the kettle to boil, or changing a nappy, for example – but where possible try different positions and give them your undivided attention, they only take a few minutes of your day.

Training positions

Initially, choose the position that feels the most effective. (This may be lying down.) Eventually you will be able to train your pelvic floor in different positions throughout the day.

- Sitting or kneeling and leaning forwards, resting on your forearms is a comfortable option. It helps you relax, feel your pelvic floor and avoid squeezing your buttocks.
- Alternatively, try lying on your side or back, sitting upright or leaning forwards, sitting cross-legged, kneeling upright or leaning forwards, standing feet and knees together, standing feet apart, walking.

Always check your posture – maintain relaxed shoulders, a long spine and a natural lumbar curve.

How many, how often, how long?

- Perform three quality pelvic-floor sets daily.
- Aim for 10 long holds or 10 quick lifts per set (although you may start with fewer and build up to more).
- Mix them up throughout the day.
- If you find them difficult early on, do just a few at a time, holding each for as long as you can. Focus on good technique and with practice and patience you will improve.
- Relax your pelvic floor between each lift for at least as long as the lift itself. Initially you may lift for three seconds, and relax for six seconds, eventually you will be able to lift for 10 seconds and relax for 10 seconds.

A few minutes each day for a lifetime of control

Pelvic-floor long holds

Starting position
- Choose from one of the positions on page 68.
- Elongate your spine, relax your neck and shoulders.

Action
- Visualise the muscular sling running from your pubic bone to your tail bone.
- Lift your pelvic floor upwards and inwards.
- Start at the back as though you are trying to control wind and then continue the contraction through to the front as though controlling your bladder.
- Make this lift and squeeze as strong as possible.
- Hold for 5 breaths, relax for 5 breaths.
- Repeat 5 times.

Modification
- You may start initially with 3 long holds, maintaining each for just 3 breaths but still resting for 5 breaths in between.

Progression
- Aim to build up to 10 long holds, sustaining each for 10 breaths and resting in between for 10 breaths.
- Continue to explore more challenging positions until eventually practising while walking.

Technique tip
- Check all other muscles are relaxed.
- Breathe normally.

Pelvic-floor quick lifts

Starting position
- Choose from one of the positions on page 68.
- Elongate your spine, relax your neck and shoulders.

Action
- Visualise the muscular sling that supported your baby in your pelvis.
- Lift your pelvic floor quickly, to maximum strength.
- Hold for 2 to 3 seconds.
- Relax for 2 to 3 breaths.
- 5 repetitions of raising and releasing, with as strong a lift as possible each time.

Modification
- Only do as many as you are able to do well, in 1 set.
- Relax for longer in between each lift.

Progression
- Aim to build up to 10 or more quick lifts in succession.
- Bring the rest phase back to 1 to 2 breaths.

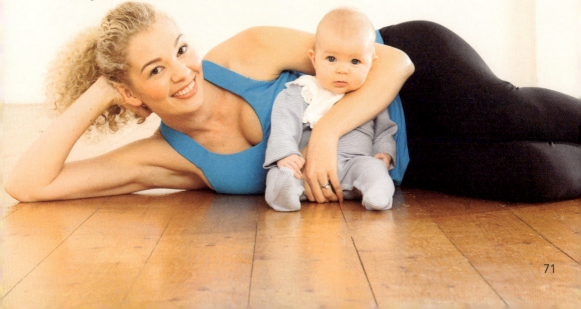

Core essentials

Training from the inside out

Strengthening your deep abdominals is your first step towards regaining your waist and provides strong and stable foundations for other exercise and your busy life as a new mum.

The transversus abdominus, in conjunction with the deep back muscle group (multifidus), the diaphragm above and the pelvic floor below, work like a low deep muscular belt, creating a cylinder of stability for your lumbar spine.

Core training, positioning and progression

Initially, core recruitment is performed while you are still. Engage your deep abdominals in the position that feels most effective. For many new mums this will be side-lying. As your core control improves you can practise in different positions such as lying, kneeling on all fours, sitting and standing, and then gradually increase the challenge by adding movement. Eventually you will incorporate core and pelvic-floor recruitment into everyday life and more advanced exercises. Your aim is to be able to recruit and maintain sound core-muscle support throughout any activity.

The foundation of movement

Core training tips

- Breathe normally.
- Elongate your spine and relax your neck and shoulders.
- Gently draw your lower abdomen towards your lower back.
- You should feel a subtle drawing inwards sensation below your navel as you recruit the deep abdominals.
- Feeling your pelvic floor lift is a sign that the muscles are working together, as they should be.
- Slowly increase the hold time. Initially you may hold for 5 breaths, then gradually build up to 10.
- As your deep abdominals get stronger you can progress to engaging and maintaining core recruitment during movement and other exercises.

The exercises on pages 74 to 81 take you through a range of core training options.

Avoid

- Holding your breath.
- Straining.
- Sucking in your waist and rib cage.
- Tensing other muscles such as your buttocks, thighs, shoulders, hands, or face.
- Shaking.
- Loss of quality movement control.

Engage your core

Practise engaging your core in the following stationary positions before progressing to the exercises involving movement:
- Lying on your side, back or front.
- Kneeling on all fours.
- Sitting.
- Standing.

Engage your core

Starting position
- Choose from one of the suggested positions above.

Action
- Lengthen your spine, place your hand below your navel.
- Gently draw inwards under your hand, taking your lower abdomen lightly towards your lower back.
- Hold this for 3 to 5 slow breaths and relax.
- Repeat 5 times.

Progressions
- Try other positions or progress to the exercises in the following section.
- Increase the hold time.

Technique tips
- Breathe normally.
- A gentle in-draw is all you need – a stronger 'sucking in' will recruit unwanted accessory muscles and compromise good core strengthening.

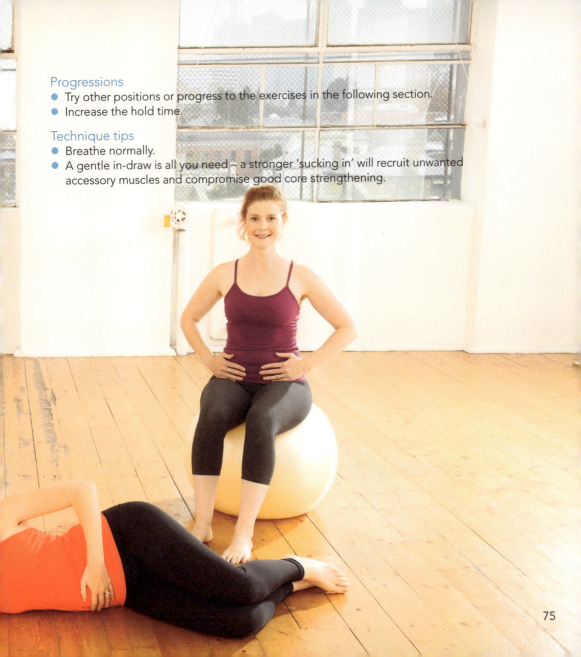

Four-point kneel

Starting position
- Kneel on all fours with your hands under your shoulders and knees under hips.
- Soften your elbows and draw your shoulder blades towards your tail bone.

Action
- Gently draw your lower abdomen towards your lower back, hold for 5 slow breaths and relax.
- Repeat 5 times.

Progressions
- Keeping your back straight, add an arm or leg raise.

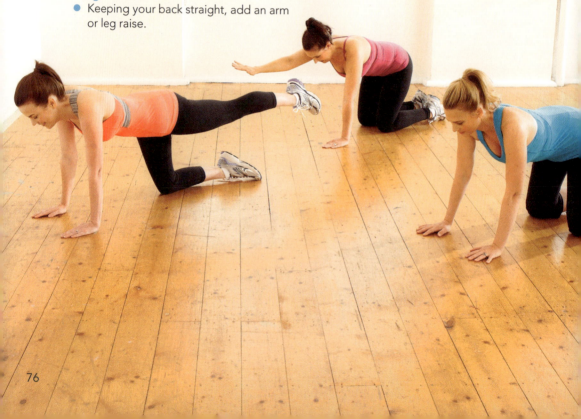

Supine leg slide

Starting position
- Lie on your back with your knees bent.
- Rest fingers on your hip bones.
- Lengthen your spine and relax your neck and shoulders.

Action
- Switch on your deep abdominals and pelvic floor.
- Slowly slide one heel along the floor to straighten your knee.
- Use your core to keep your lower back still, do not let it arch.
- Slowly slide back up and repeat on the other side.
- Repeat 5 to 10 times on each leg.

Technique tips
- Use your hands to check your pelvis does not tilt. Only go as far as your core control dictates.
- If your lower back starts to arch, slide your leg back. Work within the range you are able to control.
- Use your core to maintain neutral lumbar curve. Your other leg must remain relaxed.

Control your core and pelvis

Wall lean and reach

Starting position
- Stand with your hands on the wall a little lower than shoulder height.
- Take a step backwards, keeping your elbows slightly bent.

Action
- Lean into the wall, keeping your back and hips straight and your shoulder blades down.
- Raise one arm upwards.
- Hold this position for 5 slow breaths, relax and then repeat using other arm. 5 repetitions on each side.

Modification
- Keep both hands on the wall.
- Wall hover.

Progressions
- Step slightly further back, away from the wall.
- Add a single leg raise.
- Increase the hold time.
- Hover (page 130).

A user-friendly, effective way to boost your core control

Wall hover

A user-friendly way to train your core without overloading your back. Adding a ball provides valuable increased stability training.

Starting position
- Stand facing the wall, holding the ball at chest height against the wall (lower than your chin).

Action
- Lower your shoulders gently back and down.
- Engage your deep abdominals, drawing your lower abdomen lightly towards your lower back.
- Lean forwards, resting your forearms on the ball, keeping your back and hips straight.
- Hold this for 5 slow breaths, rest and repeat 5 times.

Modification
- Perform the hover with your forearms on the wall without the ball.
- Four-point kneeling (page 76).

Progressions
- Add a single leg raise, extending your leg behind you.
- Increase the hold time.
- Hover (page 130) or roll away (page 132).

Core control without overloading your back

Seated leg raise (ball)

Starting position
- Sit tall on a fitball.
- Place your feet slightly forwards so that your heels are under your knees and your calves are not touching the ball.

Action
- Lengthen your waist, engage your deep abdominals and settle your shoulders back and down.
- Raise one foot off the ground and extend your knee.
- Hold your knee straight for 3 breaths, slowly lower it back down then repeat on the other side.
- 5 to 10 repetitions on each leg.

Technique tips
- Maintain natural breathing and relax your shoulders downwards as you sit tall.
- Use your core to keep your back long and natural lumbar curve present.

Modification
- Sitting tall, raise your heel just off the floor, keeping your big toe on the floor for balance.
- Hold for 3 breaths then change sides.

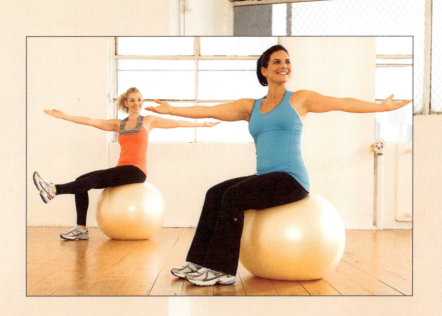

Seated spine twist

Starting position
- Sit tall on a fitball with your feet out from the ball, heels under your knees.

Action
- Lengthen your spine, engage your deep abdominals and settle your shoulders back and down.
- Raise your arms sideways to shoulder height.
- Turn your upper body slowly to one side then the other, keeping your lower back and pelvis still.
- Repeat 5 times each way.

Technique tips
- Maintain natural breathing.
- Focus on keeping your body long, your deep abdominals engaged and your shoulders relaxed.
- Keep your arms in straight alignment (as though holding a broom stick behind your upper back).

Modification
- Sit on a chair instead of a ball.

Progressions
- Placing your feet and knees together or incorporating the seated leg raise as you twist adds further core challenge.

cardiovascular fitness

Boost your fitness and lift your mood

Exercise such as walking, swimming and cycling not only raises the fitness of your heart and lungs, but also helps boost your energy for everyday life. Getting out and about with your baby or taking a little time out for you will also help to clear your head and lift your spirits. While your postnatal priority should be health, rather than dieting, there is no doubt that sensible cardio fitness will burn a few calories, enhance your endurance and put you in a healthy frame of mind but it is imperative that you are sensible and patient. Too much, too soon will impair your recovery from pregnancy and delivery. High-impact or intense cardio exercise can lead to aches and pains and be detrimental to your pelvic floor, increasing your risk of incontinence or prolapse.

Start gently, keep it low impact and only build up as your body allows.

Cardiovascular exercise guidelines

During the early weeks after delivery you can enjoy light walking and focus on smooth, controlled low-impact movement, avoiding bouncing – your pelvic floor and breasts will thank you. Prioritise good breast support and footwear and don't forget your water bottle!

As the weeks turn to months and you are feeling stronger, aim to get out for a walk most days with your baby in the pram or sling. You can then gradually increase the distance and add stroller fitness exercises within comfort. Listen to your body and cut back if you recognise signs of overdoing it.

After eight to 12 weeks, when you are well-healed and your pelvic floor and core are strong, you will be able to explore other low-impact cardio options such as swimming and fitball exercises. Eventually you can progress to low-impact aerobics, cycling and aqua fitness, but there is no rush – remember your pelvic floor.

If you are keen and ready to add intensity to your walking program, low-impact options such as power walking and hill walks are better choices than running.

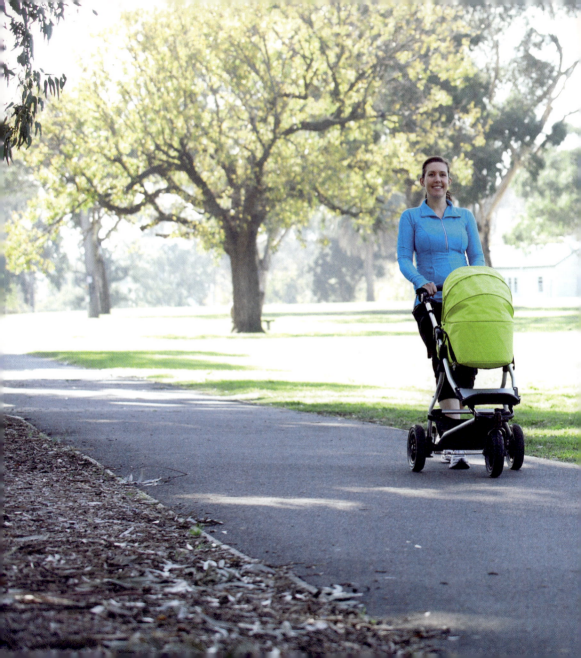

Walking

Walking is a wonderful boost to your morale as well as your fitness, as long as your joints, energy levels and pelvic floor are telling you they are ready. Start with strolls around the house or garden and gradually add a few minutes per day. Soon you will be enjoying a 15-minute walk out and about. Monitor how you are feeling and remember that every day is different.

Walking tips
- Lengthen your spine and engage your core as you walk.
- Keep your chest up, walk tall and proud.
- Avoid locking your knees and stride out within comfort.
- Find creative reminders to add some pelvic-floor strengthening – lift and hold from one lamp post to the next or add a quick lift every time you pass a tree.

After six weeks or so, assuming you are recovering well and feeling fine, you can boost your walk with one of the following:
- Add a little distance or time.
- Increase your pace – add a power walk burst every third or fourth tree or lamp post.
- Include a slope or slight hill.

When can I return to high-impact exercise?

If you have discomfort in your pelvic joints, back, breasts or any other concern you should refrain from high-impact exercise such as running, but the most significant consideration should be your pelvic floor.

You can resume high-impact exercise when you are able to do the following:
- With a full bladder, perform five star jumps or jumping jacks. Add a cough to the last two.

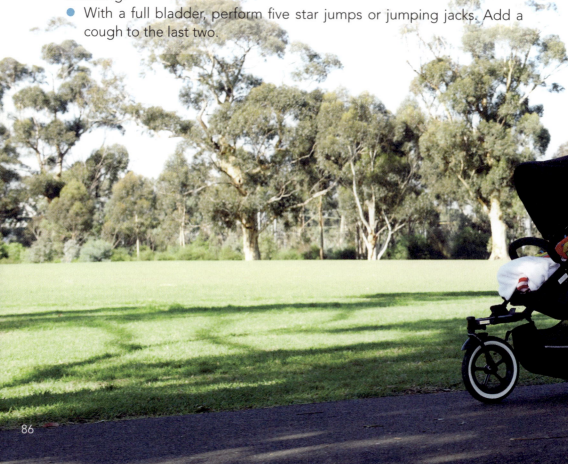

This may seem extreme, but remember that too much, too soon can lead to long-term incontinence. A little patience goes a long way towards a dry and controlled future.

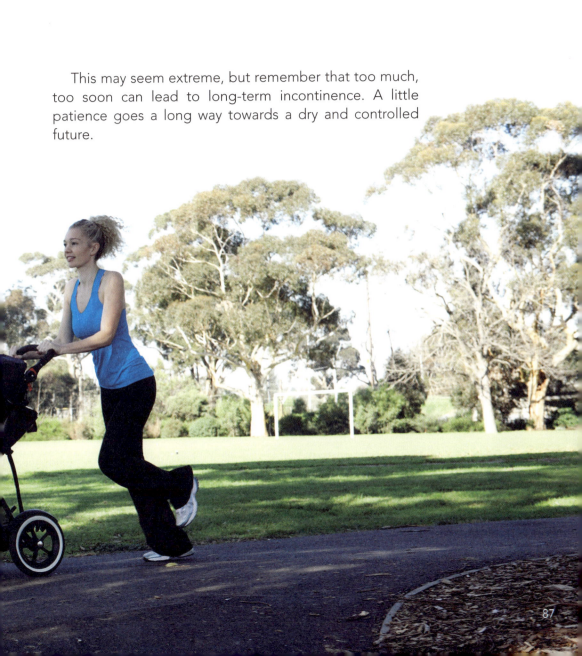

Low-impact cardio moves

Enjoy these user-friendly low-impact cardio moves in the comfort of your home – add some music for extra motivation. Perform a minute or two of each, or mix and match the moves to create your own low-impact routine. Replace these options with low-impact fitball moves if you are experiencing pelvic-joint pain (page 90).

Heel dig

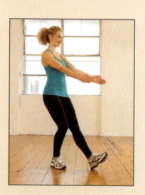

Starting position
- Stand with your feet hip-width apart.
- Squat down slightly, knees bent. Keep the weight in your heels.
- Lengthen your spine and engage your core.
- Bend your elbows by your side.

Action
- Tap alternating heels in front as you reach forwards and back.

Training tips
- Maintain the squat or carefully squat up and down with each heel dig, but do not bounce.
- Keep your back straight.

Side tap

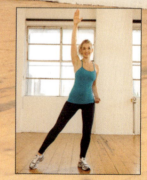

Starting position
- Stand with your feet together.
- Bend your knees to squat slightly.
- Leave your arms by your side.

Action
- Engage your core and pelvic floor.
- Tap one foot out to the side.

- Reach your arm, on the same side, upwards.
- Alternate side taps.

Training tips
- Keep the support knee slightly bent.
- Check your back stays straight.

Step touch

Starting position
- Stand feet together, arms by your sides.
- Bend your knees in a slight squat.

Action
- Step side to side as though stepping back and forth over a line, tapping the second foot beside the first.
- Reach your arms forwards and back or up and down, bending your elbows in by your sides with each step.

Training tips
- Keep your knees bent to maintain a squat with each step.
- Avoid bouncing, keep the movement smooth and controlled.

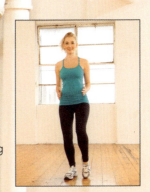

Hamstring curls

Starting position
- As step touch.

Action
- As you step side to side bend your other knee to curl your heel towards your bottom.
- Continue stepping and curling side to side.
- Reach your arms out to the side and then bend them back in with each step and curl.

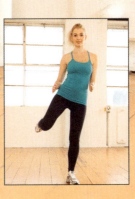

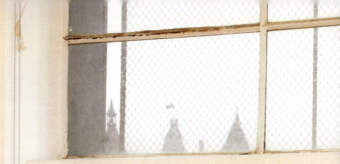

Low-impact fitball: cardio and core unite

An excellent way to add core training to your low-impact fitness and a great option for women with pelvic-joint pain.

Perform each of the following three exercises for a few minutes or mix and match to create your own fitball workout. (They each have the same start position.)

Starting position
- Sit tall on the ball, with your feet hip-width apart and slightly out so that your calves and heels are not touching the ball.
- Bend your elbows by your sides.

Fitball walk

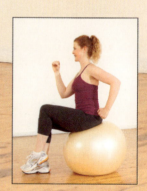

Action
- Engage your core and settle your shoulders downwards.
- Walk 2 steps forwards then back, keeping your back straight.
- Arms perform a natural walking action.

Training tip
- Keep your body upright and maintain your normal lumbar curve as you move forwards and back.

Heel dig

Action
- Tap alternating heels in front as you reach your arms forwards and back.

Training tips
- Keep your back straight.
- Each time you bend your elbows, draw them inwards to encourage upper-back strengthening.

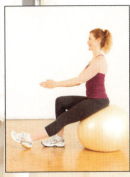

Side tap

Action
- Keep your body straight and upright as you tap alternating feet side to side.
- As you tap your foot to the side, reach the same arm upwards by your ear.

Training tips
- Keep your knee slightly bent as it taps sideways.
- Stay upright – do not let your upper body sway side to side.

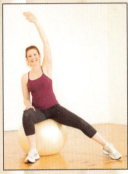

Step touch

Action
- Step a foot to the side then follow it with the second foot to tap beside the first.
- Continue stepping side to side, raising your arms to shoulder height with each step.

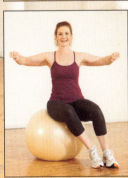

Water Fitness

Aqua exercise is a wonderful option for postnatal women. The properties of water provide assistance or resistance to your movements, allowing you to vary the workout to suit your ability and stage of recovery. Buoyancy offers relief from gravity, a superb weightless sensation, and allows an effective cardiovascular workout without straining your body.

You can enjoy water-based options once any wounds are healed but it is wise to wait until your postnatal medical check before taking the plunge.

Swimming

Start gently with your favourite stroke, stopping to take a rest whenever you feel the need.

Mix up the strokes if possible and avoid breaststroke kick if you have any pelvic-joint discomfort. Gradually add a lap or two to your swimming session and enjoy some post-swim stretches to enhance a happy, healthy posture.

Post-swim stretches include neck stretch and shoulder rolls (page 54) and chest stretch (page 172).

Alongside swimming, there are many other options for enhancing your fitness in the water.

Water walking

- Walk across the pool in waist-deep water.
- Walk forwards, backwards and sideways, using your arms to help pull you through the water.
- As your fitness improves increase the depth, speed or number of laps.

Aqua fitness

A range of moves can be performed in the water before they can on land, as the buoyancy and support minimise the impact on your body. You must still adhere to the pelvic-floor rule – the exercise is 'pelvic-floor safe' if you are able to sustain a sound pelvic-floor contraction and good bladder control throughout the activity.

In chest-deep water try a minute of each of the following:
- Jogging.
- Jumping side to side.
- Jumping forwards and back.
- Kicking alternating legs in front, pointing your toes to increase the thigh workout.
- Standing in chest-deep water raise your arms to chest height. Keeping your elbows slightly bent, push the water out to the side and then pull it back in front of you.
- Stand with your feet hip-width apart and knees slightly bent, arms reaching out in front. Push both arms to one side then the other, working your waist as you rotate your upper body.

At the pool edge:
- Hold the side of the pool and, floating on your front, engage your core and kick your legs. Focus on keeping your knees straight so you kick from your gluteals to get a good butt workout.
- Push back from the edge as though starting a backstroke race and then run back to the edge against your own current.

Deep water running:
- Using a foam noodle, aqua belt or other flotation device, perform a running or cycling action with your feet off the floor.

At the gym

There's no need to rush back to the gym with so much you can do at home and outdoors, but if, two to three months down the track, you are feeling fit and well, your core and pelvic-floor function is sound and you are ready to move on, you may choose to head to your local fitness centre.

Cycling

Cycling is an effective low-impact cardio training technique. As long as you are comfortable and you feel like it, get on an indoor bike and cycle for 10 to 15 minutes. Stick to a moderate level and avoid intense cycle classes or standing in the pedals, or riding with high resistance for many months. Have your bike correctly adjusted for your height and take care to avoid straining your joints, back or pelvic floor.

Treadmills

Treadmills are an excellent option. Start with a comfortable five to 10-minute walk, and build up gradually to a faster walk or by adding an incline. Keep it low-impact until you have excellent pelvic-floor control.

Group exercise classes

There is a vast selection of group fitness classes nowadays. Classes vary from mind/body to extreme and challenging boot-camp styles. When you feel ready to return to a class and you have checked all the criteria, take a moment to consider which style is right for you. Choose low-impact over high, and avoid classes that involve heavy weights or extreme moves.

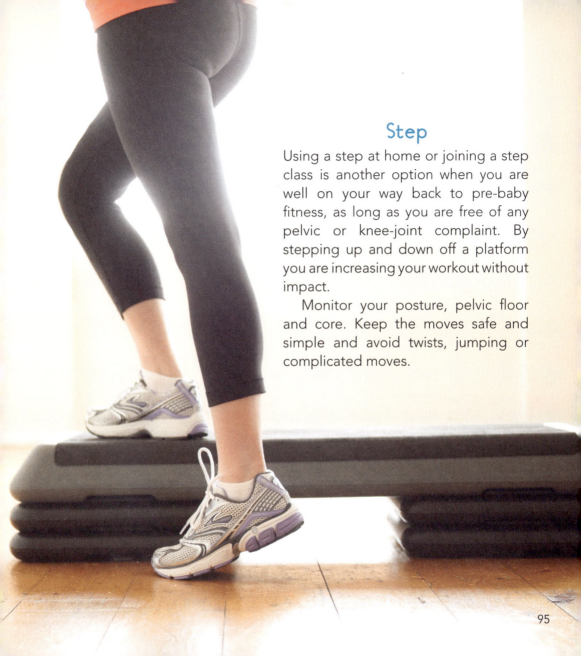

Step

Using a step at home or joining a step class is another option when you are well on your way back to pre-baby fitness, as long as you are free of any pelvic or knee-joint complaint. By stepping up and down off a platform you are increasing your workout without impact.

Monitor your posture, pelvic floor and core. Keep the moves safe and simple and avoid twists, jumping or complicated moves.

Strengthen and tone

Muscle conditioning

- Will help you regain your strength, muscle tone and fitness.
- Assists healthy weight management.

Strengthening outer muscles such as quadriceps or biceps must go hand in hand with inner-muscle support. Always engage your core in conjunction with outer-muscle exercises. Remember, if you are unable to sustain the deep-muscle support, decrease the challenge.

For healthy, upright posture balance your workout front and back, training opposing muscle groups such as biceps and triceps, hamstrings and quadriceps, and be sure to include plenty of back strengthening.

Inner and outer muscles working in harmony

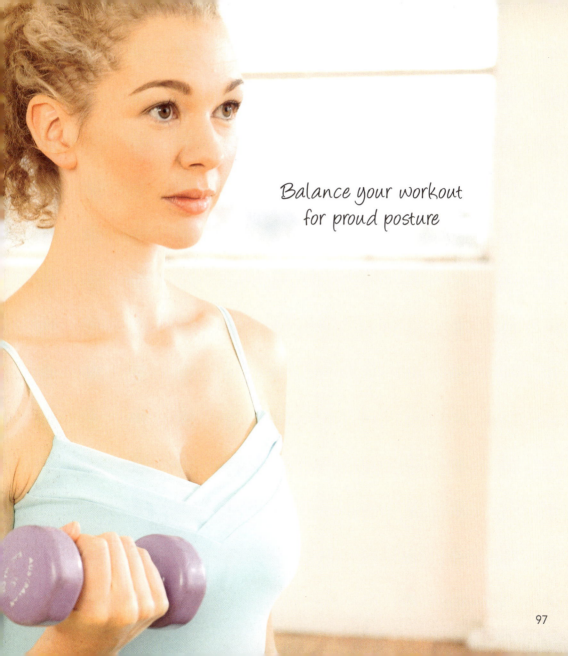

Balance your workout for proud posture

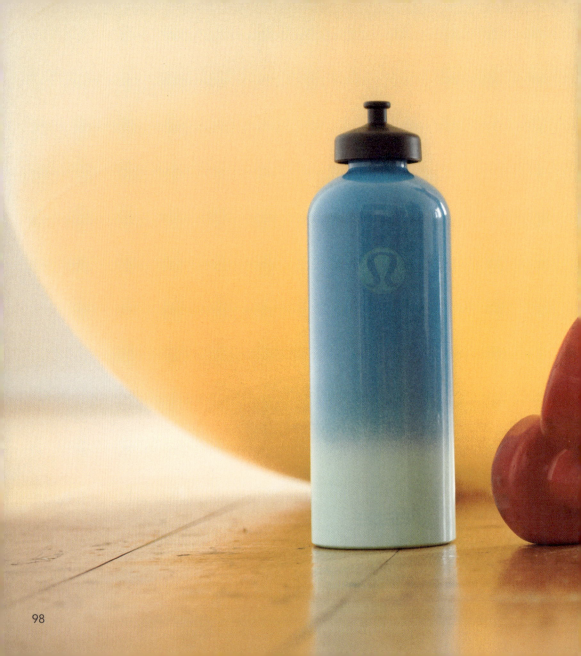

Strength training: how much, how heavy?

Low-resistance, high-repetition strength exercises are ideal for postnatal women. Heavy weights place too much stress on your back, abdominals, joints and pelvic floor. When using strength-training equipment, such as hand weights or exercise bands, the resistance is correct if you can perform 10 to 15 repetitions, while breathing normally and maintaining excellent posture and smooth-flowing motion. Aim to feel your muscles working by the last few repetitions, but if you lose form or feel you are straining you should lighten the load. Progress carefully, always ensuring full range of movement and excellent technique.

Start with 10 repetitions and when you feel ready add a second set of 10. Build up to two sets of 15 and, as you get stronger, add a third set or increase your weights slightly.

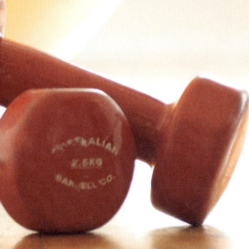

Every strength exercise has a complementary stretch. You may choose to stretch after each exercise or complete a combination of stretches at the end of your workout. Either way, ensure you make time to include stretching in your routine, your body will thank you.

Strength-training tips

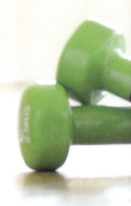

- Always engage your core and pelvic floor first.
- Select a resistance that allows you to perform one set of 10 to 15 repetitions with good form.
- Add a second and third set as you get stronger.
- Modify and progress to suit your individual ability.
- Focus on fine form and perfect posture.
- Breathe normally.
- Include plenty of back-conditioning exercises to help strengthen your posture.
- Avoid overload – holding your breath, shaking, losing form or compromised posture are signs you need to decrease the load or number of repetitions.
- Expect to commence strength training later and progress more gradually if you have had a caesarean section, abdominal separation or continence concerns.

When can I return to strength training?

You can commence core and pelvic-floor recruitment when your baby is just a few days old but it is best to avoid lifting anything heavier than your baby for at least six weeks.

You can resume light strength exercises that do not strain or load your back, abdominals or pelvic floor when you feel your core and pelvic floor are strong and working well. This may be weeks or months after delivery, everyone is different. Later you will add stronger and more challenging moves – for most this should not be until your baby is 10 to 12 weeks old.

Tips for checking you are ready for strength exercise

- Engage your core and pelvic floor then perform the exercise in question.
- If you are unable to maintain a strong core and pelvic-floor muscle contraction to the end of the exercise, you do not yet have the foundation support for that move.
- Once you are able to maintain core recruitment, perform as many repetitions as your core control dictates.

Upper-body strength training

Strengthen your upper body for lifting, life and perfect posture.

Biceps curls

Starting position
- Stand tall or sit on a fitball.
- Elongate your spine and relax your shoulders.
- Arms straight by your sides, hold hand weights, palms facing forwards.

Action
- Engage your core and pelvic floor.
- Slowly bend your elbows, bringing your hands towards your shoulders.
- Lower them back down with control.
- 15 repetitions x 2 sets.

Technique tips
- Keep your back straight.
- Keep your elbows tucked in close by your sides.

Modification
- Lighten the load.

Progression
- Increase the load.
- If sitting on a fitball, for increased core challenge add alternating seated leg raise (page 80).
- Combine biceps curls with wall squat (page 115) or standing (narrow) squat (page 114).

Stretch
- Open your heart (page 57).

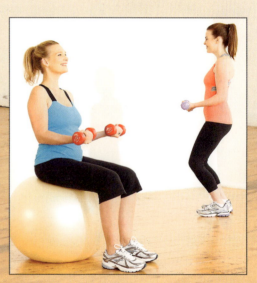

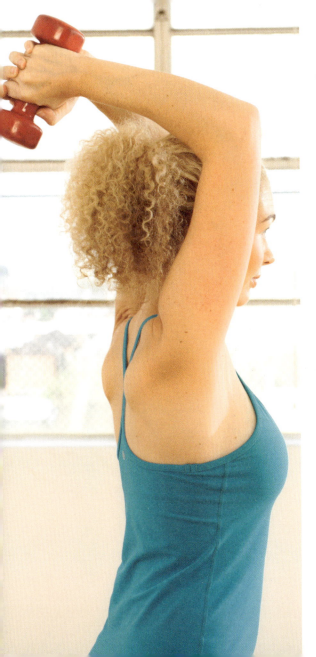

Triceps press

Starting position
- Sit on a fitball or stand tall.
- Hold one weight behind your head.
- Bend elbows and tuck in so they are close to your head.
- Lengthen your spine, engage your core and draw your shoulder blades downwards.

Action
- Extend your arms to press the weight upwards.
- Bend your elbows to lower it back down.
- 15 repetitions x 2 sets.

Technique tip
- Avoid shrugging your shoulders.

Modification
- Lighten the load.

Progression
- Increase the weight or perform a third set.
- If seated on a ball add an alternating seated leg raise (page 80).

Stretch
- Triceps stretch (page 172).

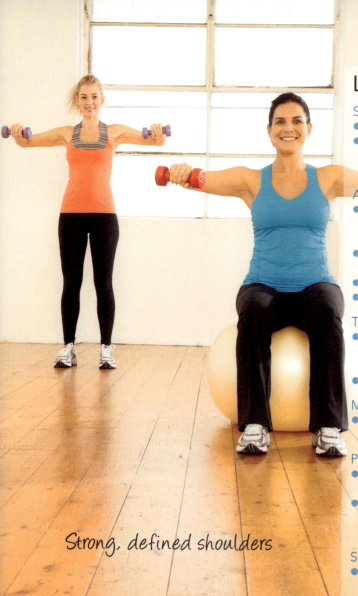

Strong, defined shoulders

Lateral raise

Starting position
- Sit or stand tall.
- Hold hand weights with your elbows bent to 90 degrees and tucked in by your sides.

Action
- Lengthen your spine, draw your shoulder blades downwards and engage your core.
- Raise your arms sideways to shoulder height.
- Lower them slowly.
- 15 repetitions x 2 sets.

Technique tips
- Keep your arms aligned so that your hands and weights go no higher than your elbows.
- Avoid shrugging your shoulders.

Modification
- Decrease the repetitions, load or perform one set only.

Progression
- Increase the load or perform a third set.
- If seated on a ball add an alternating seated leg raise (page 80).

Stretch
- Neck stretch and shoulder rolls (page 54).

Narrow row

Starting position
- Sit on a fitball or stand tall.
- Hold hand weights with your elbows bent by your sides.

Action
- Elongate your spine and engage your core.
- Reach forwards.
- Bend your arms backwards, drawing your elbows back and in.
- 15 repetitions x 2 sets.

Technique tips
- Keep your posture straight and strong.
- Consciously draw your shoulder blades down and inwards as you bend your elbows back, to emphasise the back-strengthening component of this exercise.

Modification
- Decrease the load or repetitions or perform 1 set only.

Progression
- If seated on a ball, add alternating seated leg raise (page 80).
- If standing, add a narrow-based squat (page 114).

Stretch
- Open your heart (page 57).

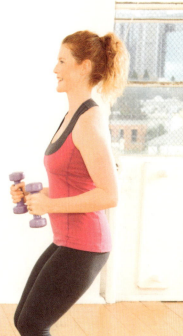

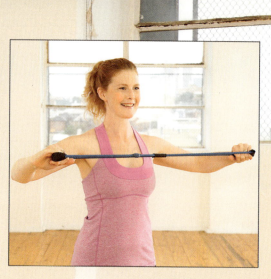

Wide row

Starting position
- Sit on a fitball or stand tall with arms in front of chest, elbows almost straight.
- Hold an exercise band in front of you at chest height.
- Hands shoulder-width apart with slight tension on the band.

Action
- Engage your deep abdominals and pelvic floor.
- Draw your shoulder blades inwards and downwards as you bend your elbows, taking your hands wide to stretch the band.
- Slowly release the tension as you return to the starting position.
- 15 repetitions x 2 sets.

Technique tip
- Feel the muscles between your shoulder blades working.

Modification
- Lengthen the band slightly.
- Perform fewer repetitions or only 1 set.

Progression
- Shorten the band slightly.
- Add an extra set.
- Add alternating leg raise (seated) if sitting on the ball (page 80).

Stretch
- Upper-back stretch (page 173).

Upper-back strength for perfect posture

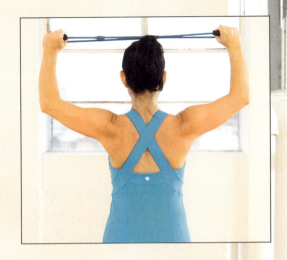

Lat pull-down

Starting position
- Sit on a fitball or stand tall.
- Hold an exercise band up high, slightly forwards rather than directly above your head.
- Your arms should be angled up and forwards.

Action
- Lengthen your spine, engage your core and settle your shoulders back and down.
- Bend your elbows and pull your hands down and outwards to stretch the band.
- Feel the muscles in your back drawing your shoulder blades downwards.
- 15 repetitions x 2 sets.

Technique tips
- Your hands should go wider than your elbows.
- Engage your core and keep your back strong and stable.

Modification
- Perform the exercise without the band, using a strong technique to allow you to feel the muscles in your back working.
- Perform 15 repetitions x 1 set, or 10 repetitions x 2 sets.

Progression
- Slightly shorten the band.
- Add a third set.

Stretch
- Side stretch (page 175) and upper-back stretch (page 173).

Chest press

Strengthen your core, gluteals and pecs.

Using the ball is an advanced exercise for mums who are strong and fully recovered.

The floor option is a lighter alternative for mums earlier on.

Starting position
- Sit on a fitball, hold hand weights, resting them on your thighs.
- Round your back then carefully walk your feet out and roll down, using your elbows to support you.
- Keep rolling until your shoulder blades are on the ball.
- Lower you head to the ball and straighten your back.
- You should have a straight body and be supported by the ball through your head, neck and shoulder blades, with your neck in line with your spine.
- Your heels should be under your knees.
- Lift your pelvis by squeezing your gluteals.
- Engage your deep abdominals to support your lower back.
- Prepare for the chest press, taking your bent elbows out to be level with your shoulders and your forearms and hands pointing upwards.

Action
- Engage your core and pelvic floor.
- Push your heels into the ground and squeeze your buttocks to keep your pelvis raised.

- Press the weights upwards to be end to end above your chest.
- Lower them back slowly, taking your hands wider than your elbows.
- 15 repetitions x 2 sets.
- Drop your bottom slightly to rest between sets.

Technique tips
- Keep your back straight – do not let your hips drop, nor your spine arch.
- To sit back up, lower your hips, put your weights on the ground then rest your elbows on the ball to assist control. Put your chin on your chest and walk your feet backwards, rolling yourself to an upright sitting position.

Modification
- Perform the chest press lying on the floor with your knees bent.

Progression
- Add a third set.
- Bring your knees and feet together for added core challenge.

Stretch
- Back stretch and roll (page 58).

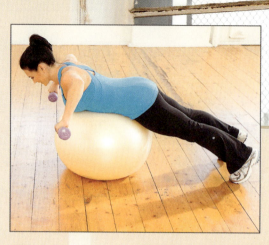

Prone wide row

Starting position
- Lie prone (face downwards) over the ball.
- Lean through the balls of your feet, pushing your heels towards the ground.
- Raise your chest slightly up off the ball (using your back muscles).
- Look at the floor, keeping your neck in line with your spine.

Action
- Hold light hand weights end to end in front of the ball, just off the floor.
- Draw your shoulder blades towards your tail bone.
- Bend your elbows as you raise your arms to take the hand weights upwards and outwards in a wide arc.
- Lower them slowly.
- 15 repetitions x 2 sets.
- Rest, kneeling, on the floor between sets.

Technique tips
- Lean firmly through your feet (do not just balance on your toes).
- Focus on squeezing your shoulder blades together.

Modification
- Perform this action with lighter weights.
- If you find this hard work for your back or uncomfortable because you have had a caesarean you may prefer to do the wide row (page 106).

Progression
- Slowly raise one leg then the other with each row.
- Add a third set.

Stretch
- Upper-back stretch (page 173).

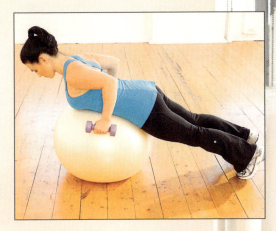

Prone triceps

Starting position
- Lie prone over the ball, hold hand weights by your hips and bend your elbows, keeping them high and close to your body.

Action
- Slowly straighten your elbows to press the weights towards the ceiling.
- Bend your elbows to lower the weights back down.
- 15 repetitions x 2 sets.
- Rest, kneeling, on the floor between sets.

Technique tip
- Keep your elbows high and tucked inwards, as though they are hooked over a pole that is running across your back.

Modification
- Perform the move without weights.
- Decrease the reps or sets.
- If you find this hard work for your back or uncomfortable because you have had a caesarean you may prefer the upright triceps press (page 103).

Progression
- Add a third rep or slightly increase your weights.

Stretch
- Triceps stretch (page 172).

Breaststroke

Starting position
- As exercise on page 110, then place hands close together just in front of your chest.

Action
- Reach your arms forwards, then out and around in a wide arc taking your hands to your hips and then together again in front, ready to repeat the breaststroke action.
- 15 repetitions x 2 sets.
- Rest, kneeling, off the ball between sets.

Technique tip
- Hold your chest up off the ball and keep your neck in line with your spine.

Modification
- 'Swim' with one arm at a time, the other hand resting on the ball.
- If lying prone on the ball is uncomfortable, especially if you had a caesarean delivery, replace with wide row (page 106).

Progression
- Add an alternate leg raise to bring your butt into the picture and further strengthen your back.

Stretch
- Upper-back stretch (page 173).

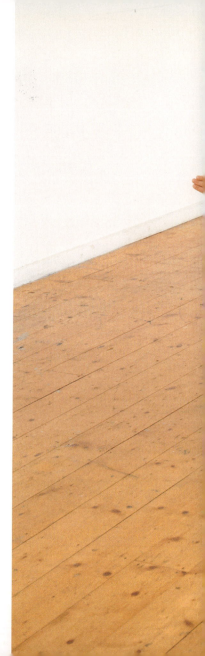

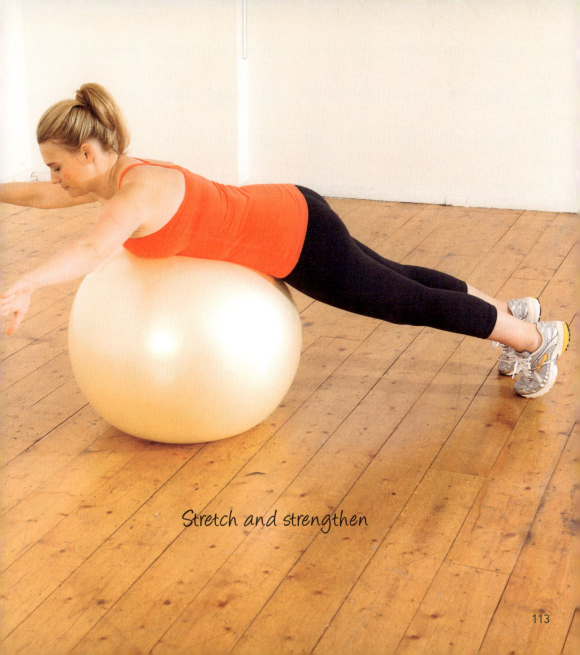

Stretch and strengthen

113

Lower-body strength training

Narrow squat

Starting position
- Stand tall with your feet hip-width apart.
- Settle your shoulders back and down.

Action
- Lift your pelvic floor and draw your lower abdomen inwards to switch on your core.
- Keep the weight in your heels as you slowly bend your knees and hips (as though you are sitting down).
- Push your heels into the ground, and slowly stand back up, tucking your tail bone in and under.
- 15 repetitions x 2 sets.

Technique tips
- Keep your weight in your heels to protect your knees.
- The lower you squat the stronger the move.

Modification
- Seated leg raise on chair or ball (page 80).

Progression
- Holding hand weights, add a narrow row (page 105), reaching forwards as you squat down and bending your elbows back and inwards as you stand up.

Stretch
- Prone quads stretch (page 176).

Tone your thighs, butt and back

Wall squat

Starting position
- Stand with the ball between you lower back and the wall.
- Bend your knees to squat down into a seated position.
- Adjust your feet so that your heels are under your knees and you can just see your toes.
- Engage your core and check that your back is straight.
- Move the ball so that it is supporting you from your tail bone to your middle back.

Action
- Engage your core and pelvic floor.
- Slowly stand and 'sit', rolling the ball up and down the wall.
- 15 repetitions x 2 sets.

Technique tips
- Keep your back straight and vertical – avoid leaning forwards or back.
- Keep your body weight in your heels to protect your knees.

Modification
- Do not squat as deeply.
- Decrease your reps and sets.
- Seated leg raise, ball (page 80).

Progression
- Using hand weights, add a controlled biceps curl as you squat.
- Add a third set.

Stretch
- Prone quads stretch (page 176).

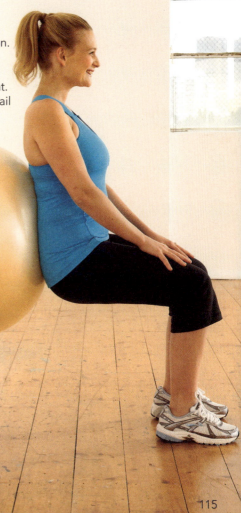

Ball bridge

Starting position
- Sit on a fitball, round your back then carefully walk your feet out and roll down until your elbows touch the ball.
- Keep rolling until your shoulder blades are supported.
- Lower your head to the ball and straighten your back.
- Check your body is straight and your head, neck and shoulder blades are on the ball.
- Your heels should be under your knees.

Action
- Draw your lower abdomen towards your lower back to recruit your core.
- Slowly lower and raise your hips.

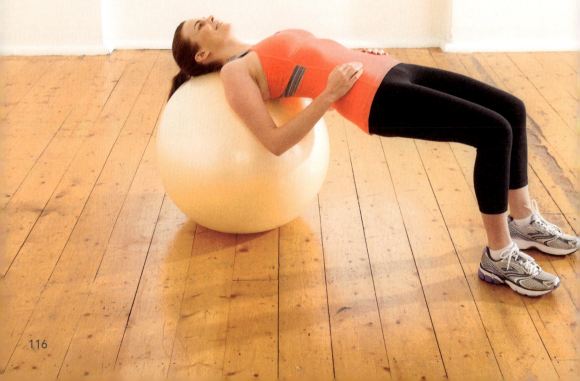

- Press your heels into the floor and squeeze your gluteals each time you raise your pelvis to the neutral position.
- 15 repetitions x 2 sets.
- Lower your hips and rest your elbows on the ball between sets.

Technique tips
- Use your gluteals and core together.
- Do not arch your back.

Modification
- Baby bridge (page 162).

Progression
- Bring your feet and knees together.
- Perform a third set.

Stretch
- Back stretch and roll (page 58) or supine gluteals stretch (page 177).

An advanced option for your back and butt

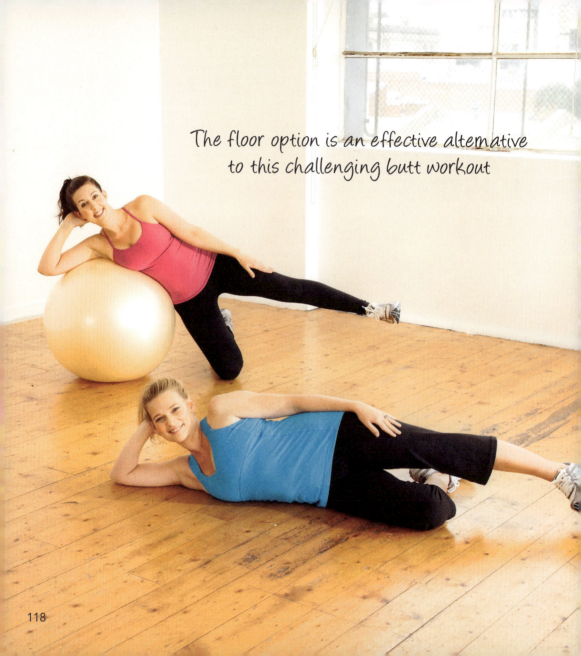

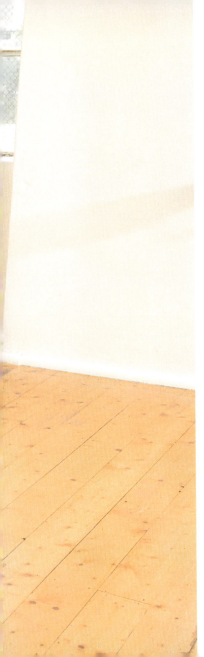

Thigh side lift

Starting position
- Kneel with the ball firmly against your thigh.
- Lie sideways over the ball.
- Extend your outside leg.
- Slide the supporting knee away slightly to allow you to lean into the ball.
- Rest your head in your hand.

Action
- Engage your core and pelvic floor.
- Straighten your leg with your knee and foot pointing straight ahead.
- Raise and lower your leg slowly.
- 15 repetitions x 2 sets.
- Rest off the ball between sets.

Technique tips
- Squeeze your leg straight.
- Lean into the ball.
- Keep the ball and your pelvis still and stable.

Modification
- Lying on the floor.

Progression
- Add a third set.

Stretch
- Supine gluteals stretch (page 177).

Swim kick

Starting position
- Lie prone over the ball with your hands resting lightly on the floor.
- Roll forwards and lift your feet to extend your legs in line with your body.
- Using your back muscles, find the balance point where you need very little or no weight on your hands.

Action
- Perform a slow, straight-leg kicking action, working from your buttocks.
- 15 kicks on each leg x 2 sets.

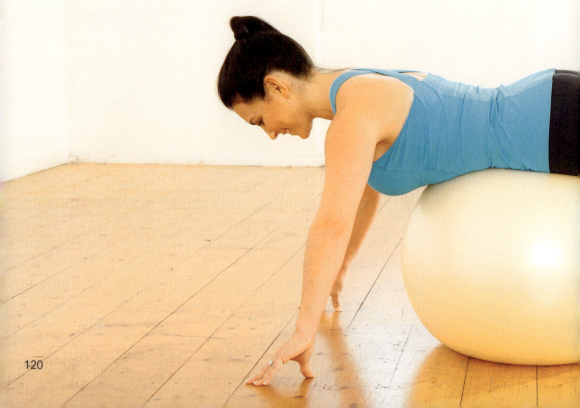

Technique tips
- Keep your knees straight.
- Look at the floor to avoid straining your neck.
- The less you lean on your hands, the more you strengthen your back.

Modification
- Swim kick on the floor.
- Baby bridge (page 162).
- Four-point kneel with leg raise (page 76).

Progression
- Kick with no weight on your hands, just resting lightly on your fingertips.
- Perform a third set.

Stretch
- Kneeling back-and-butt stretch (page 175).

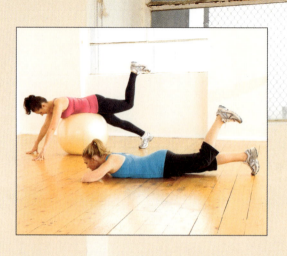

Hamstring curl

Starting position
- Lie prone on the ball.
- Lean your weight through the ball of one foot, the other leg extended to hip height.

Action
- Bend your knee, bringing your heel towards the ceiling.
- Work with muscle tension as though you are curling and straightening against resistance.
- 15 repetitions on one leg, rest off the ball, then 15 on the other leg.

Technique tips
- Keep your neck in line with your spine by looking at the floor.
- The less you lean through your hands the more you strengthen your back.

Modification
- Lying on the floor is an excellent alternative (see photo above).
- Four-point kneel with leg raise may be more comfortable if you have had a caesarean (page 76).

Progression
- Increase the reps or repeat a second set on each leg.

Stretch
- Kneeling back-and-butt stretch (page 175).
- Supine hamstring stretch (page 176).

Hamstring lift and roll

Starting position
- Lie on the floor with your arms relaxed by your sides.
- Ensure the backs of your heels are resting on top of the ball.

Action
- Engage your core and pelvic floor.
- Press your heels down into the ball as you raise your hips off the floor.
- Roll the ball towards you until your knees are bent above your hips.
- Roll the ball away.
- Lower your hips back to the floor.

Technique tips
- Keep your feet flexed back towards you.
- Ensure the soles of your feet stay off the ball.
- Push down with the back of your heels into the ball.
- Keep your neck, shoulders and arms relaxed.

Modification
- Baby bridge (page 162).
- Raise and lower your hips only.

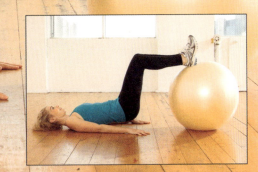

Progression
- Taking your arms off the floor will increase the core challenge.

Stretch
- Supine hamstring stretch (page 176).

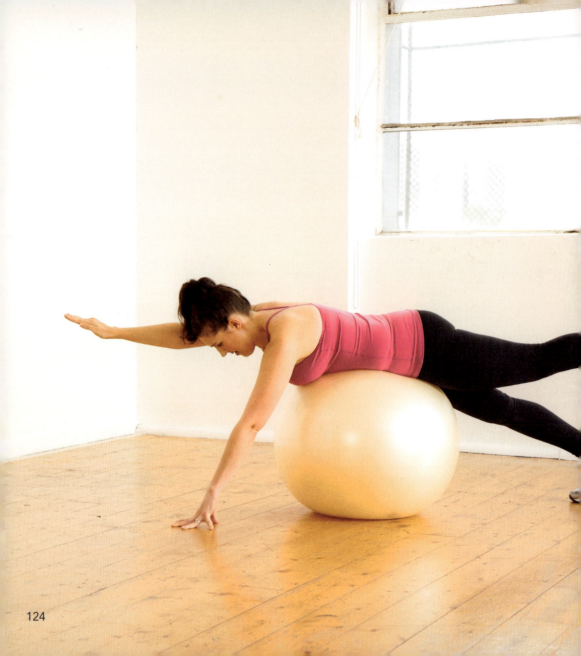

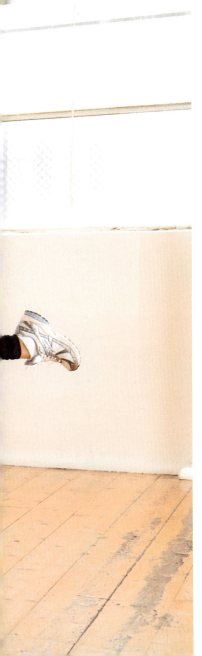

Prone arm and leg raise

Starting position
- Prone on the ball.
- Lean into the balls of your feet and rest your hands lightly on the floor.
- Engage your back muscles to lift your chest off the ball.

Action
- Raise one arm and the opposite leg.
- Stretch from top to toe, holding for 3 breaths.
- Lower slowly and repeat on the other side.
- 15 repetitions on each side.

Technique tips
- Use your back muscles to hold your chest up, with minimal weight on your floor hand.
- Stabilise your body by taking plenty of weight into the foot that is on the floor.
- Look at the floor to relax your neck.

Modification
- Raise one limb at a time.
- Four-point kneeling plus arm and leg raise will be more comfortable if you have had a caesarean section (page 76).

Progression
- Hold each limb raise for 5 breaths.
- Add a second set on each side.
- If your back is strong try raising two arms and one leg.

Stretch
- Kneeling back-and-butt stretch (page 175).

Abdominals

Abdominal curls are often the first exercises new mums are keen to get back to and yet they should be one of the last. You can eventually return to abdominal curls when your baby is 12 weeks or older, but it is helpful to remember that they do not help you lose weight or flatten your tummy.

Ab curls and crunches work the outer abdominal muscle layers and should be considered an advanced postnatal exercise because they create an increased abdominal pressure, which means they can compromise core, pelvic floor and abdominal separation recovery if performed too early.

Abdominal curls can be included in a well-balanced training program but they must not be performed until your core and pelvic floor are strong and fully functional, your abdominal separation is resolved, you are free of any hint of back or neck pain and you are completely recovered if you had a caesarean delivery. Core exercises (page 74 to 81) and low-load abdominal exercises, such as pelvic tilt (page 128) and seated rotation (page 129) are excellent options you can enjoy in the meantime.

Correct abdominal-curl technique involves all the abdominal layers. Always engage the deep muscles and pelvic floor first, to stabilise the spine, before the outer rectus abdominus or obliques to perform the curl itself. (See page 135.)

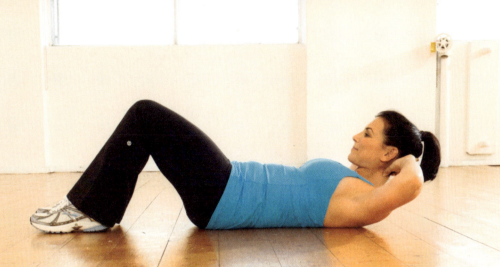

To test your readiness for abdominal curls:
- Lie on your back with your knees slightly bent and your feet on the floor.
- In-draw your deep abdominals and lift your pelvic floor.
- Raise your head and shoulders off the floor to recruit your outer abdominals.
- Breathe normally.
- Lower your head and shoulders to relax your outer abs.
- Relax your core and pelvic floor.

Your deep abdominals and pelvic floor must be able resist the increased intra-abdominal pressure and stabilise throughout the curl. If your outer abdominal wall domes or you lose the deep-abdominal and pelvic-floor muscle recruitment when you try a curl, you are not yet ready. Continue core and pelvic-floor exercises for another few weeks before trying again.

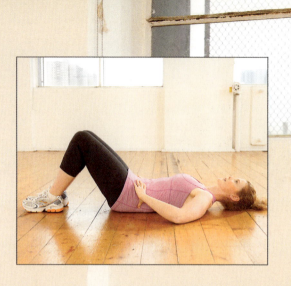

Pelvic tilt

Starting position
- Lie on your back with your knees slightly bent, feet on the floor.
- Rest your hands lightly on your hip bones.
- Elongate your spine and relax your neck and shoulders.

Action
- Draw your lower abdomen towards your lower back and lift your pelvic floor.
- Visualise your outer abdominals running from your ribcage to your pelvis.
- Use these outer abs to tilt your pelvis towards your ribs, rounding your lower back and lifting your tail bone off the floor.
- Roll your pelvis back to the natural lumbar position.
- 15 repetitions x 2 sets.

Technique tips
- Relax your legs and use your abdominals not your legs to tilt your pelvis.
- Breathe normally.

Modification
- Practise engaging your core without the pelvic tilt.

Progression
- Perform pelvic tilt in other positions such as sitting, standing and kneeling on all fours.

Stretch
- Supine rotation (page 174).

Seated rotation

Starting position
- Sit tall on a fitball, feet out in front, hip-width apart.
- Lengthen your spine and engage your core and pelvic floor.

Action
- Rotate your upper body side to side as you reach one arm then the other across your body.

Technique tips
- Think of rotating your upper body on a stable base.
- Lengthen your waist and keep your pelvis and legs still.

Modification
- Seated core (page 75).

Progression
- Bring your feet and knees together or add alternating leg raise to increase the core challenge.

Stretch
- Pelvic circles (page 152).

Hover

Starting position
- Lie on your front, propped on your forearms.
- Draw your shoulder blades towards your tail bone.
- Raise your feet and shins off the floor by bending your knees.

Action
- Engage your core.
- Raise your midsection off the floor until you are weight-bearing through your thighs and forearms.
- Attain a straight alignment from your shoulders to your knees: draw your shoulder blades downwards, engage your deep abdominals and check you are straight at the hips.
- Hold the hover for 5 slow breaths.
- Relax and repeat x 5 sets.

A more advanced exercise for women who are well-recovered and feeling strong

Technique tips
- By bending your knees you can weight-bear through your thighs rather than your kneecaps.
- Check you are not shrugging your shoulders, rounding your upper back, arching your lower back or bending at the hips.

Modification
- Wall hover (page 79).

Progression
- A more challenging hover is on your forearms and feet.
- Roll away (page 132).

Stretch
- Kneeling back-and-butt stretch (page 175).

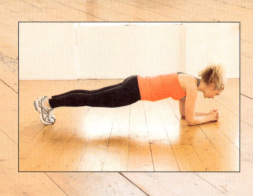

Roll away

Starting position
- Kneel upright with your hands resting on the ball, arm's-length away.

Action
- Draw your shoulder blades downwards, your lower abdominals inwards, lift your pelvic floor and lightly engage your gluteal muscles.
- Roll the ball away as you incline forwards to end up leaning on your forearms on the ball.
- Keep your shoulders down, your back and hips straight.
- Hold this for 5 slow breaths, relax and repeat x 5 sets.

Technique tips
- Lifting your feet off the floor allows you to rest on your thighs rather than your kneecaps.
- Do not let your upper back slouch, your shoulders shrug, your lower back sway or your bottom stick out.

Modification
- Wall hover with fitball (page 79).

Progression
- Increase the hold time or number of repetitions.

Stretch
- Kneeling back-and-butt stretch (page 175).

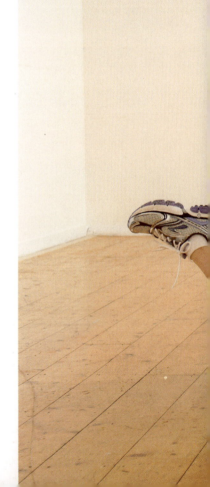

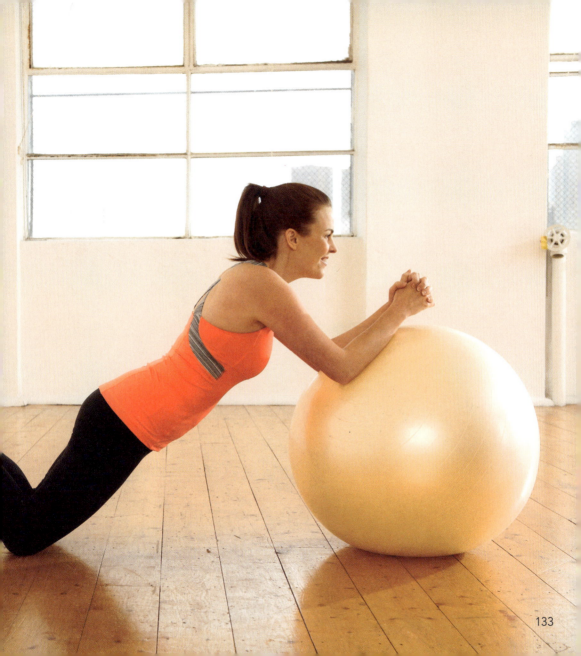

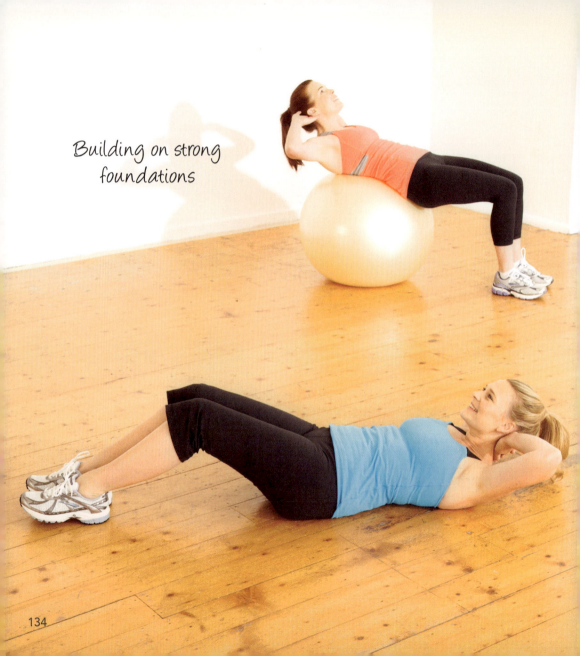

Building on strong foundations

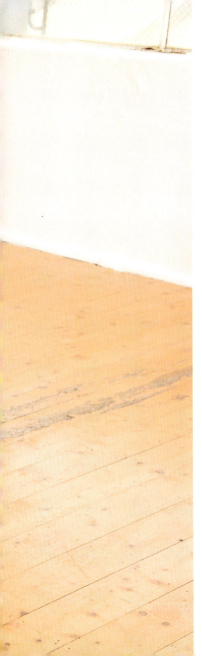

Abdominal curls

Starting position
- Lie on your back with your knees slightly bent and feet on the floor.
- Place fingers behind your ears to support the weight of your head.

Action
- Engage your core, drawing your lower abdomen towards the floor and lifting your pelvic floor towards your heart.
- Curl your head and shoulders off the floor slowly.
- Hold for one breath and then slowly roll back down.
- 10 repetitions x 2 sets.

Technique tips
- Breathe normally.
- Relax your thigh and hip muscles.
- Keep your elbows back.
- Allow the weight of your head to rest in your hands but do not lift with your arms, use your abs.

Modification
- Pelvic tilt (page 128) or supine leg slide (page 77).

Progression
- If you are feeling very strong you can try an abdominal curl on the ball, being sure your tail bone to lower back is well supported by the ball.

Stretch
- Prone extension (page 177).

Obliques curls

Starting position
- Lie on your back with your knees slightly bent and feet on the floor.
- Place fingers behind your ears to support the weight of your head.

Action
- Engage your core, drawing your lower abdomen towards the floor and lifting your pelvic floor towards your heart.
- Reach one arm up and across your body.
- Reach up and over as you slowly lift your head and shoulders off the floor, raising one shoulder more than the other to turn your upper body.
- Hold for 1 breath and then slowly roll back down.
- 10 repetitions then rest before repeating on the other side.

Technique tips
- Breathe normally.
- Relax your thigh and hip muscles.
- Allow the weight of your head to rest in your hands but do not lift with your arms, use your abs.
- Keep your arm extended across your body. Do not swing it back and forth. Use muscle not momentum.

Modification
- Seated rotation (page 129).

Progression
- If you are feeling very strong you can try obliques curls on the ball, being sure your tail bone to lower back is well supported by the ball.

Stretch
- Supine rotation (page 174).

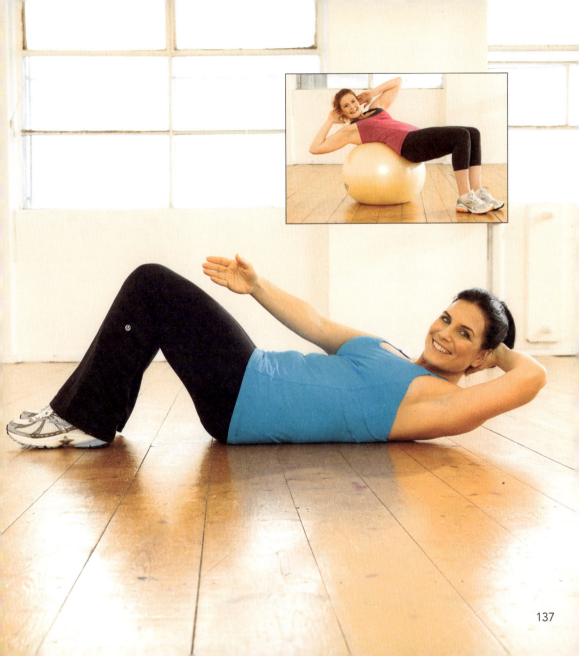

Stroller fitness

Getting out and about is a great way to lift your spirits as well as your fitness. We all know walking is a fabulous form of exercise for postnatal women, but there is plenty more you can do to boost strength and well-being while you are enjoying being with your baby, your friends, a change of scenery and some fresh air.

When walking with the pram or sling:
- Stand tall.
- As your fitness and recovery progress stride out a little more.
- Aim to feel like you are exercising but still be able to talk.
- Avoid locking your knees.
- Do not over-grip the pram.

Interesting ways to include pelvic-floor and core strengthening

- Lift your pelvic floor as you pass a lamp post then hold it strong and tight until the next lamp post. Relax for three lamp posts and repeat.
- Gradually increase the distance you can walk while holding your pelvic floor at maximal lift.
- Consciously lengthen your spine and draw your deep abdominals towards your lower back every time you pass a tree.

Enjoy the following user-friendly exercises in the park. They can also be added to your home-based exercise repertoire and can be done with or without the pram.

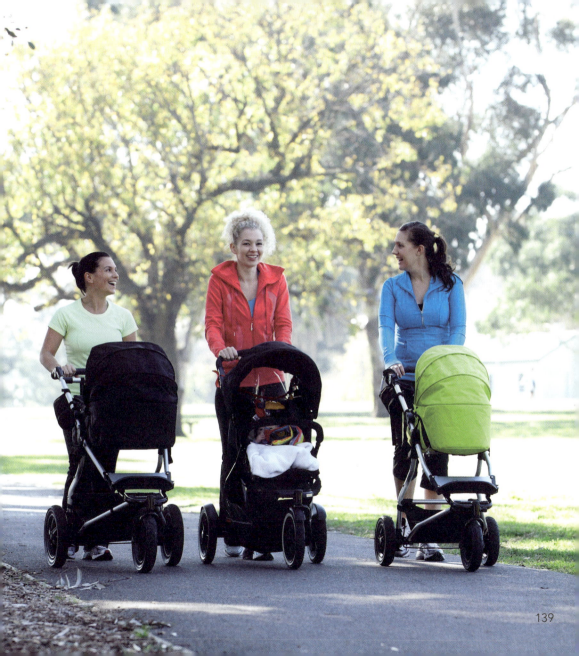

Calf raise

Starting position
- Stand tall, resting your fingers lightly on the pram.
- Feet hip-width apart.

Action
- In-draw your lower abdomen and lift your pelvic floor.
- Raise your heels so you are up on the balls of your feet.
- Lower slowly.
- Continue raising up and down.
- 15 repetitions x 2 sets.

Technique tips
- Keep your knees soft (slightly bent).
- Use your hands for balance only, fingers light on the pram.

Stretch
- Calf stretch. See inset photo below – step one foot as far back as you can, pushing your heel into the ground as you bend your front knee and lunge slightly forwards. Hold for 10 slow breaths and repeat on the other leg.

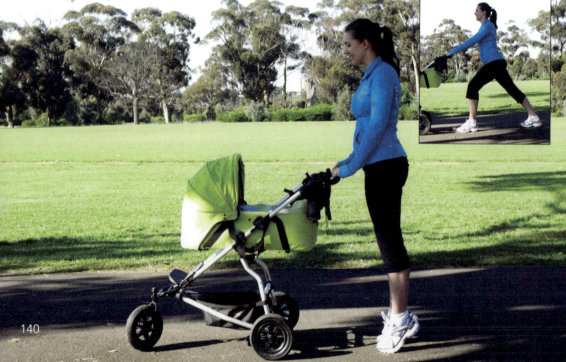

Squat and row

Starting position
- Stand tall, both hands resting lightly on the pram.
- Feet hip-width apart.

Action
- Engage your core and pelvic floor.
- Squat down, bending your knees as you do so.
- Simultaneously push the pram away.
- Push your heels into the ground and squeeze your buttocks as you stand back up and bring the pram back towards you.
- 15 repetitions x 2 sets.

Technique tips
- Keep the weight in your heels to protect your knees.
- Your upper body will incline forwards as you squat down, but keep your back straight.

Modification
- Seated leg raise, chair (page 145).

Progression
- Squat and leg extension (page 142).
- Squat and side leg lift (page 143).

Stretch
- Quads stretch (as per page 176 but in standing position, using one hand on your pram for balance).

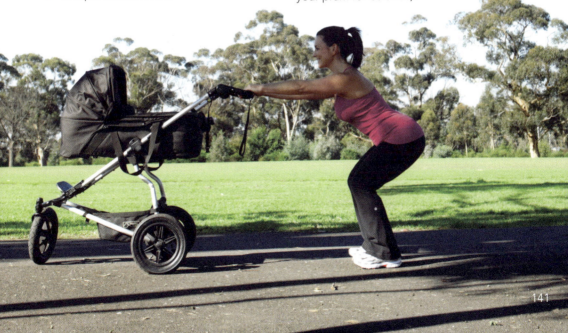

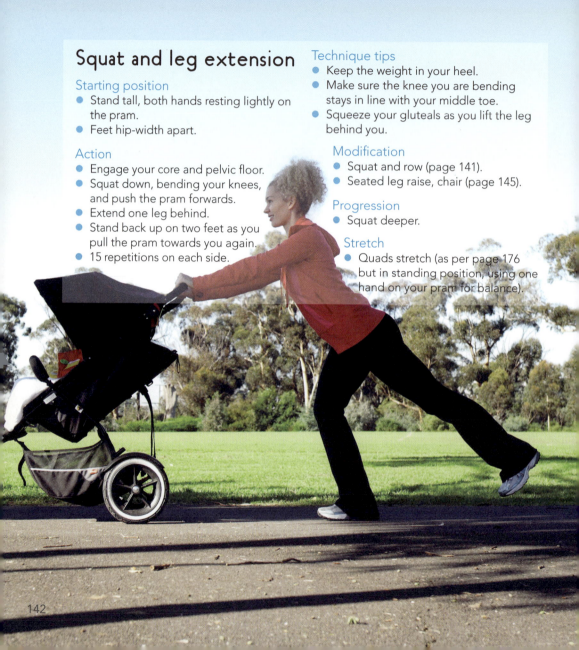

Squat and leg extension

Starting position
- Stand tall, both hands resting lightly on the pram.
- Feet hip-width apart.

Action
- Engage your core and pelvic floor.
- Squat down, bending your knees, and push the pram forwards.
- Extend one leg behind.
- Stand back up on two feet as you pull the pram towards you again.
- 15 repetitions on each side.

Technique tips
- Keep the weight in your heel.
- Make sure the knee you are bending stays in line with your middle toe.
- Squeeze your gluteals as you lift the leg behind you.

Modification
- Squat and row (page 141).
- Seated leg raise, chair (page 145).

Progression
- Squat deeper.

Stretch
- Quads stretch (as per page 176 but in standing position, using one hand on your pram for balance).

Squat and side leg raise

Starting position
- Stand tall, beside your pram, one hand resting on the handle.
- Ensure your feet are just a little apart.

Action
- Engage your core and pelvic floor.
- Squat down, bending your knees, and push the pram away.
- Raise your outside leg sideways.
- Return to standing as you pull the pram back towards you.
- 15 repetitions on each side.

Technique tips
- Keep your back straight, avoid leaning sideways.
- Tense the muscles in the thigh of your lifting leg and keep your foot and knee pointing straight ahead.

Modification
- Squat and row (page 141).
- Seated leg raise, chair (page 145).

Progression
- Increase the repetitions or sets.

Stretch
- Quads stretch (as per page 176 but in standing position, using one hand on your pram for balance).

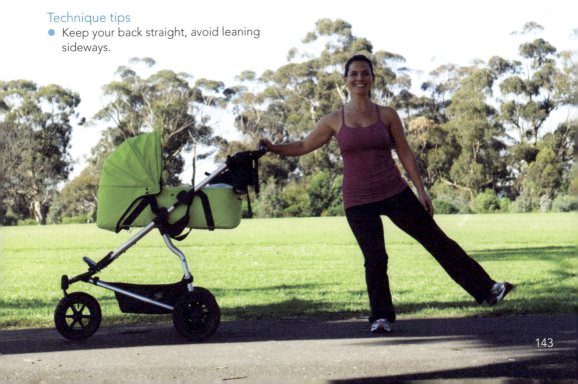

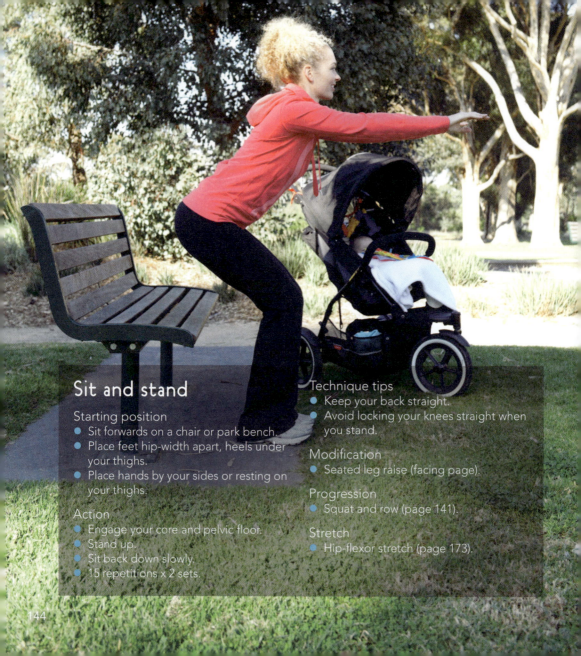

Sit and stand

Starting position
- Sit forwards on a chair or park bench.
- Place feet hip-width apart, heels under your thighs.
- Place hands by your sides or resting on your thighs.

Action
- Engage your core and pelvic floor.
- Stand up.
- Sit back down slowly.
- 15 repetitions x 2 sets.

Technique tips
- Keep your back straight.
- Avoid locking your knees straight when you stand.

Modification
- Seated leg raise (facing page).

Progression
- Squat and row (page 141).

Stretch
- Hip-flexor stretch (page 173).

Seated leg raise (chair)

Starting position
- Sit tall on a chair or bench, with your back unsupported.

Action
- Lengthen your spine and engage your core.
- Extend one knee to raise your foot to knee height.
- Squeeze your thigh muscles for 3 breaths.
- Lower back down and swap legs.
- Alternate 15 on each side, rest and perform a pelvic-floor lift then repeat a second set.

Technique tip
- Keep your back straight and strong.

Progression
- Sit and stand (facing page).

Stretch
- Hip-flexor stretch (page 173).

Take it easy on your knees as you strengthen your thighs

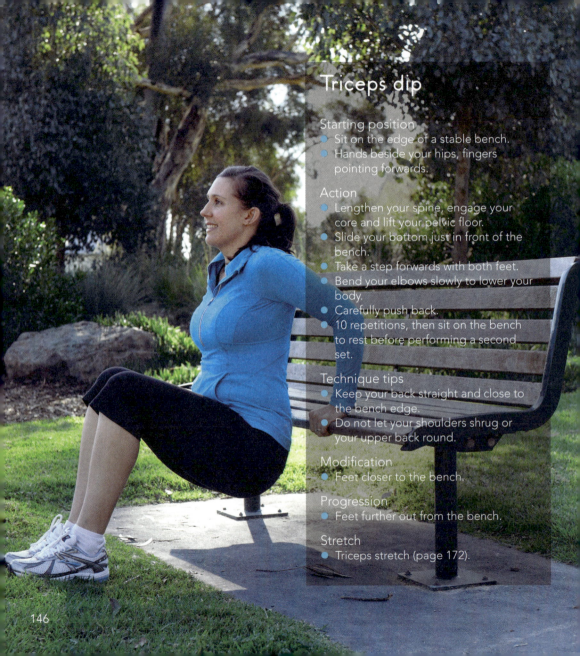

Triceps dip

Starting position
- Sit on the edge of a stable bench.
- Hands beside your hips, fingers pointing forwards.

Action
- Lengthen your spine, engage your core and lift your pelvic floor.
- Slide your bottom just in front of the bench.
- Take a step forwards with both feet.
- Bend your elbows slowly to lower your body.
- Carefully push back.
- 10 repetitions, then sit on the bench to rest before performing a second set.

Technique tips
- Keep your back straight and close to the bench edge.
- Do not let your shoulders shrug or your upper back round.

Modification
- Feet closer to the bench.

Progression
- Feet further out from the bench.

Stretch
- Triceps stretch (page 172).

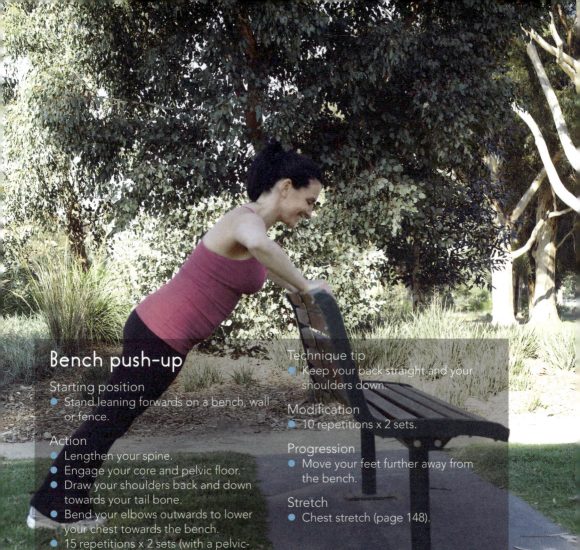

Bench push-up

Starting position
- Stand leaning forwards on a bench, wall or fence.

Action
- Lengthen your spine.
- Engage your core and pelvic floor.
- Draw your shoulders back and down towards your tail bone.
- Bend your elbows outwards to lower your chest towards the bench.
- 15 repetitions x 2 sets (with a pelvic-floor lift while you rest in between).

Technique tip
- Keep your back straight and your shoulders down.

Modification
- 10 repetitions x 2 sets.

Progression
- Move your feet further away from the bench.

Stretch
- Chest stretch (page 148).

Chest stretch

Starting position
- Stand beside your pram.
- Rest your hand on the handle.

Action
- Turn away from the pram to stretch across your chest and shoulder.
- Hold for 10 slow breaths and repeat on the other side.

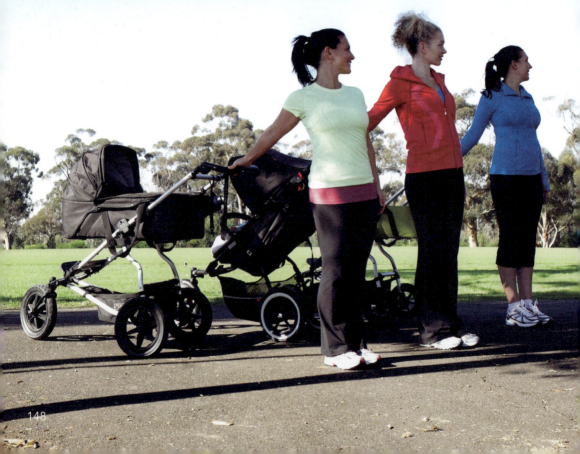

Side stretch

Starting position
- Stand beside your pram, resting one hand on the handle.

Action
- Reach your arm up and over to stretch your arm and side.
- Hold for 10 slow breaths then turn to stretch the other side.

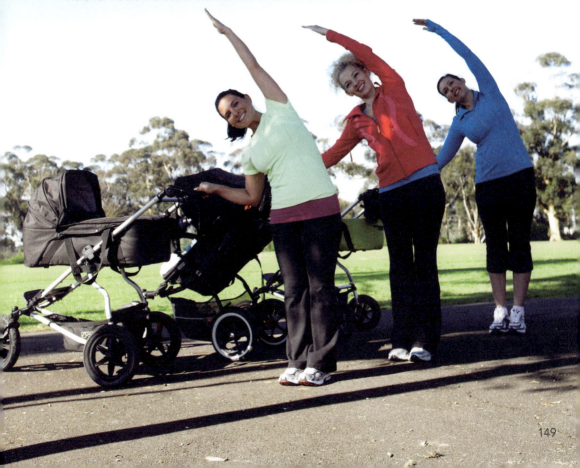

Fitness time for you,
precious time for you both

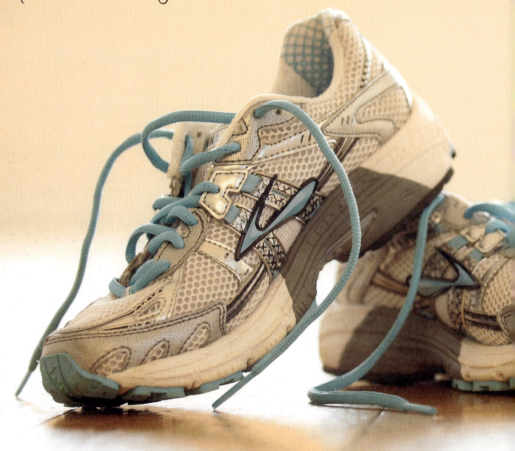

Mum-and-bub Workout

Working out with your baby is time effective and a great way to interact and play with your baby while you boost your own strength and fitness for motherhood.

Many of these exercises require a degree of postural and head control on your baby's part, so you may find them easier when your baby is two to three months or older. This is a good time for you to be starting these strengthening moves, as well.

Enjoy the following activities with your baby. They can also be performed without your baby and added to your overall workout repertoire.

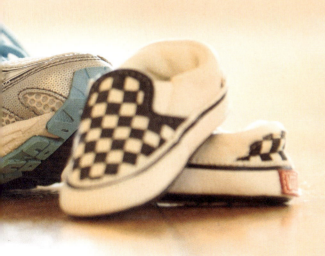

Pelvic circles

Starting position
- Sit tall on a fitball with your baby on your lap.

Action
- Roll the ball and pelvis in a slow, smooth circle.
- Keep your upper back still, rotating from the waist down.
- 10 circles each way.

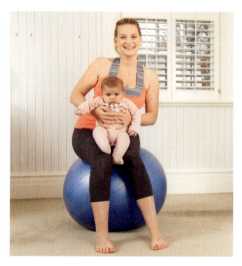

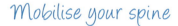

Seated bounce

Starting position
- Sit tall on a fitball with your baby supported on your lap.

Action
- Bounce gently up and down for a minute or two.
- Keep your back straight and your feet on the floor, the weight in your heels.

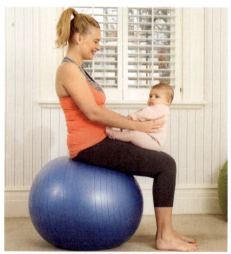

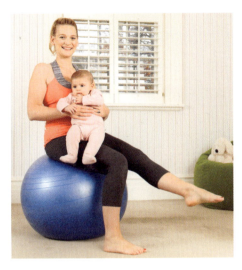

Seated leg raise (fitball)

Starting position
- Sit tall on a fitball with your baby supported on your lap.

Action
- Keeping your back straight raise one foot, lower back down slowly, then repeat with the other.
- Maintain the natural curve in your lumbar spine.
- 15 raises on each leg.

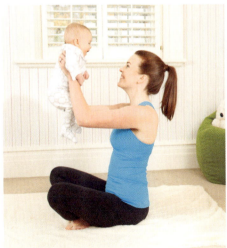

Baby fly

Starting position
- Sit or stand holding your baby, facing towards you.

Action
- Engage your core and lift your pelvic floor.
- Slowly lift and lower your baby.
- 10 repetitions x 2 sets.

Four-point kneeling with limb raise

Starting position
- Kneel on all fours over your baby.

Action
- Draw your lower abdomen towards your lower back.
- Reach one arm forwards, hold for 5 slow breaths then relax and repeat on the other side.
- Now reach one leg out behind, hold for 5 slow breaths and repeat on the other side.

Technique tip
- Keep your back straight and level.

Progression
- Combine one arm and the opposite leg.

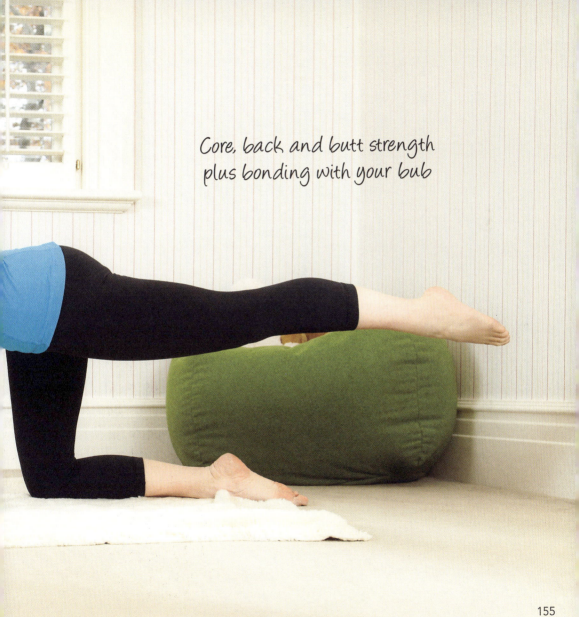

Core, back and butt strength plus bonding with your bub

All-fours triceps and lats push-back

Starting position
- Kneel on all fours over your baby.
- Hold a hand weight with your elbow bent higher than your lower back and tucked in close to your side.
- Engage your core and pelvic floor.

Action
- Extend your elbow to straighten your arm and push the weight upwards.
- Lower back slowly.
- 10 repetitions of each exercise, then change arms.
- Now holding your arm by your hip, palm upwards and elbow just slightly bent, push your hand gently up and down to work your lats x 10 small lifts on each arm.

Stretch
- Triceps stretch (page 172).

Hug and squat

Starting position
- Stand with your feet hip-width apart.
- Hold your baby securely facing towards you.

Action
- Engage your core and pelvic floor.
- Squat down and lift your baby away from your chest.
- Stand back up and hug your baby to your heart.
- 10 repetitions x 2 sets.

Technique tip
- Keep your back straight and the weight in your heels.

Stretch
- Prone quads stretch (page 176).

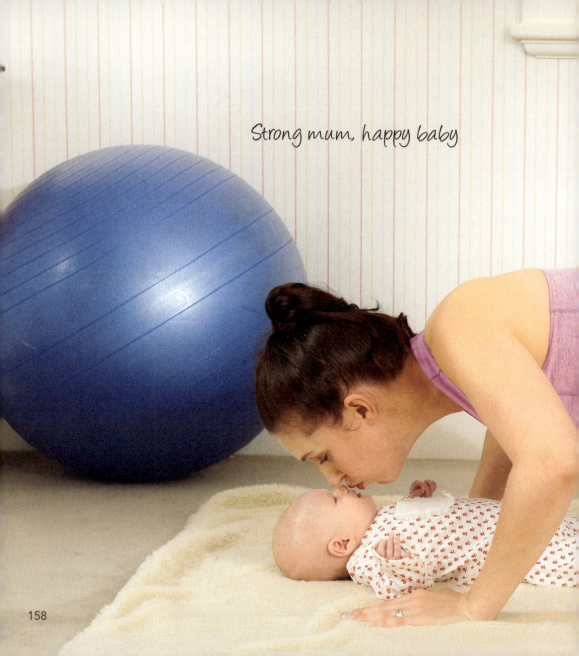

Push-up kisses

Starting position
- Kneel over your baby.

Action
- Engage your core and pelvic floor.
- Bend your elbows to lower your body towards your baby then push slowly back up.
- 10 baby kisses x 2 sets.

Technique tip
- Keep your back straight.

Progression
- Walk your knees further back and perform the push-up with straight hips.

Stretch
- Kneeling back-and-butt stretch (page 175).

Supine leg lower

Starting position
- Lie on your back with your baby supported and sitting on your tummy.
- Engage your deep abdominals.
- Raise one leg then the other, bringing your hips and knees to a 90-degree angle.

Action
- Slowly lower one foot to touch the floor lightly.
- Bring it back up and repeat on the other side.
- Lower one leg then the other 10 times x 2 sets.

Technique tip
- Do not let your lower back arch off the floor – use your deep abdominals to maintain neutral spine position.

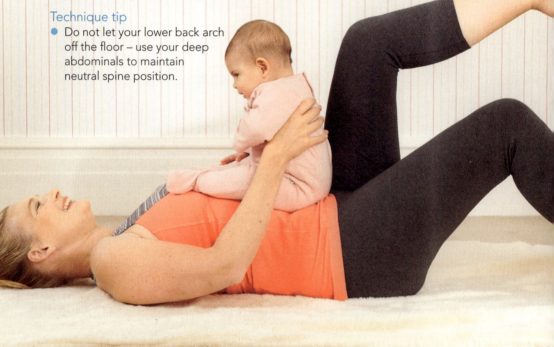

Baby curls

Starting position
- Lie on your back with your baby supported and sitting on your tummy.
- Slightly bend your knees, with your feet on the floor.

Action
- Engage your deep abdominals and pelvic floor.
- Slowly raise and lower your head and shoulders off the floor.
- 10 repetitions x 2 sets.

Technique tip
- Keep your core engaged and legs relaxed.

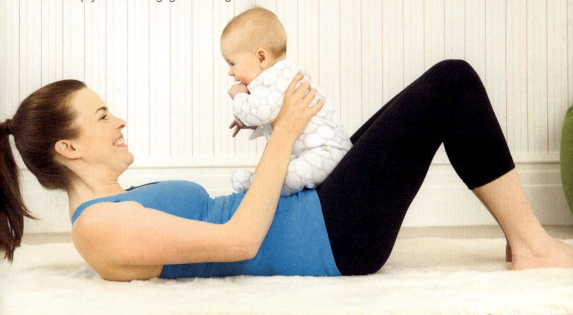

Baby bridge

Starting position
- Lie on your back with your baby supported and sitting on your tummy.
- Bend your knees, keeping your feet on the floor and heels in line with your bottom.

Action
- Engage your core and pelvic floor.
- Squeeze your gluteals and push your heels into the ground as you slowly raise your hips, taking your baby for a ride.
- Lower slowly.
- 15 repetitions x 2 sets.

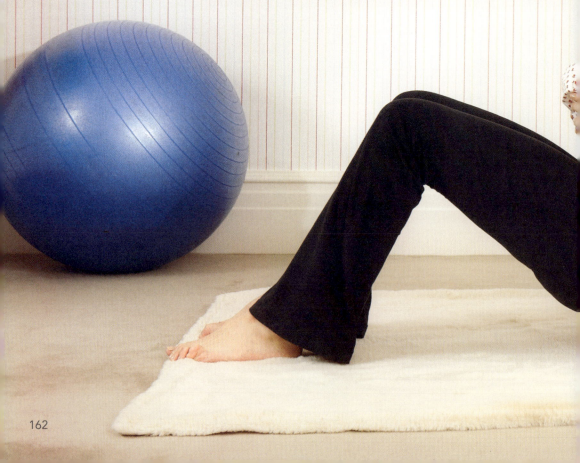

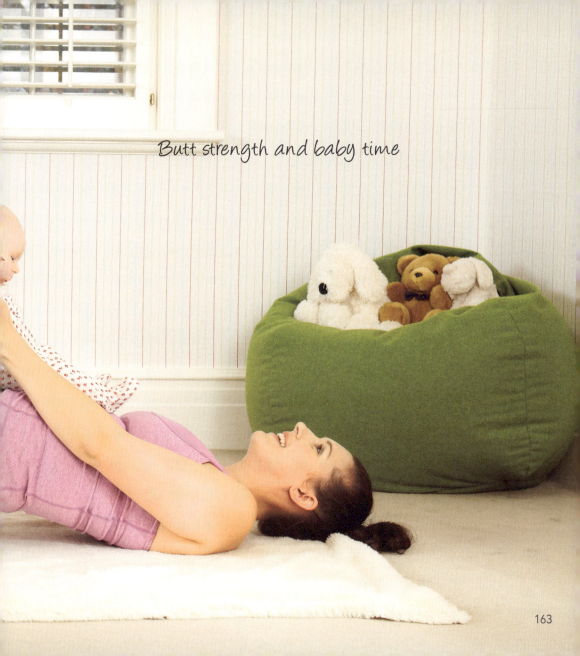

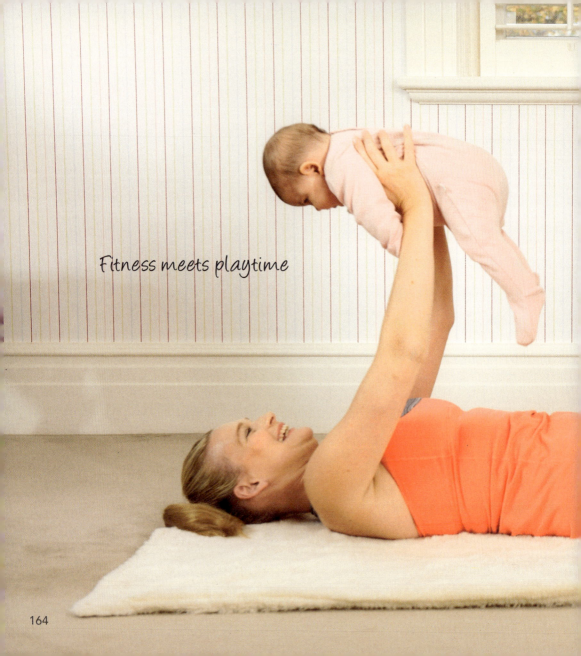

Fitness meets playtime

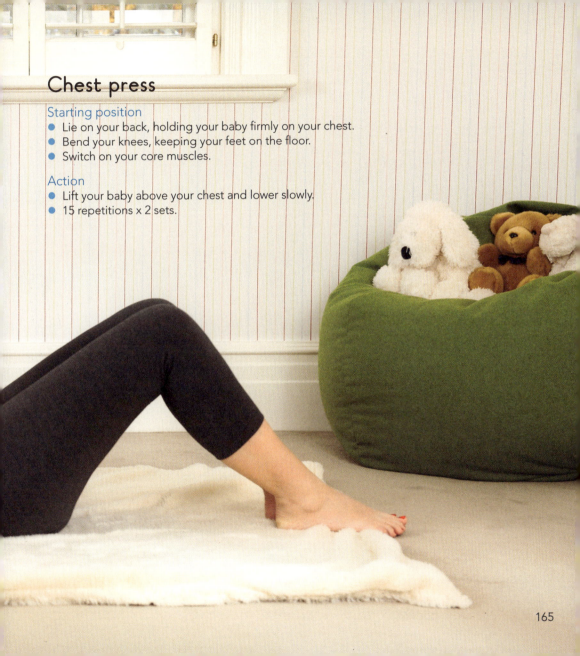

Chest press

Starting position
- Lie on your back, holding your baby firmly on your chest.
- Bend your knees, keeping your feet on the floor.
- Switch on your core muscles.

Action
- Lift your baby above your chest and lower slowly.
- 15 repetitions x 2 sets.

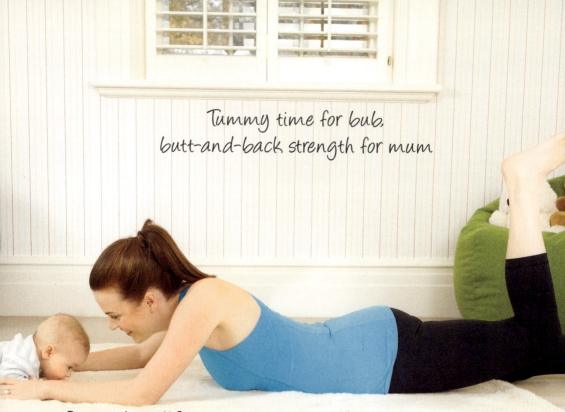

Tummy time for bub, butt-and-back strength for mum

Prone leg-lift

Starting position
- Both you and your baby lie on your fronts, facing each other.
- Rest on your forearms.

Action
- Bend one knee to a 90-degree angle.
- Squeeze your gluteals and lift your knee up off the floor.
- Hold for 3 breaths as you encourage your baby to look up at you.
- 15 repetitions on each leg.

Technique tip
- Keep your hip on the floor as you raise your thigh.

Tummy time

Starting position
- Both you and your baby lie on your fronts, facing each other.
- Place your hands on the floor under your shoulders.

Action
- Raise your chest off the ground, providing light assistance as required through your arms.
- Encourage your baby to extend too.
- 5 repetitions x 3 sets.

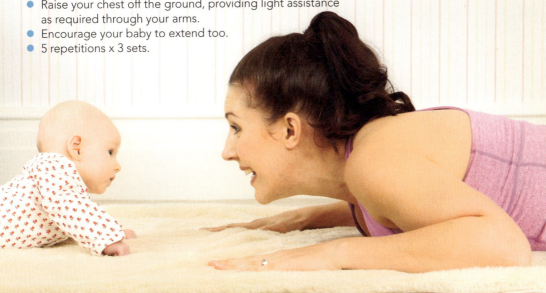

Back strengthening for mum and bub

Relaxation

Teaching your mind to become calm and quiet is invaluable for new mums – among the busy hours of your day a touch of relaxation can go a long way. The more you practise relaxation the more powerful a tool it can be. Just five or 10 minutes can become a rejuvenating and refreshing break. Take the time to put your feet up, breathe and allow peace to flow over your body, while giving yourself permission to do absolutely nothing.

Explore a range of relaxation techniques:
- Sit or lie comfortably.
- Consciously allow your breath to become slower and deeper.
- Enjoy quietness or peaceful, relaxing music.
- Focus on relaxing each body part as you breathe, starting at your feet and slowly working your way up to your neck, shoulders and face.

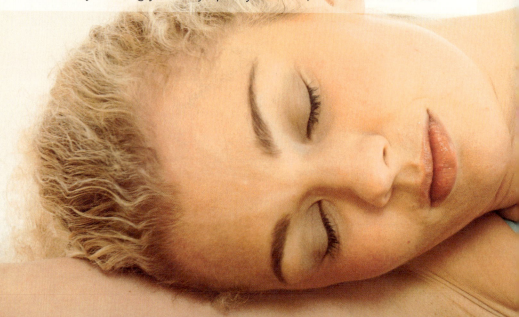

- Visualise a calming location, such as a beach, rainforest or mountainside. (See below.)
- Indulge in some aromatherapy.
- Listen to guided relaxation recordings.

Create your own visualisation

- Make yourself comfortable in a quiet, warm place.
- Settle in, close your eyes and consciously slow your breath.
- Take your mind to a place that you find relaxing, calm, quiet and peaceful. (This place can be real or imaginary.)
- Make yourself comfortable there.
- Continue to breathe slowly.
- Look around this place and take in the details of all the elements that make it special and beautiful.
- The only thing you ever do when you are here is relax.
- Breathe slowly, allowing the tension to leave and a softness and lightness move through your body.
- Enjoy your calm and precious place.

Finishing
- When you are ready to leave, start to move your hands and feet gently.
- Gradually move and stretch as you come back to here and now.
- As you take an awakening stretch and return rejuvenated, remember that you can go to this special place whenever you like.

Stretching

Stretching and relaxation are important elements of any health and fitness program.

Tight muscles can cause discomfort, postural imbalances and injury. Gentle stretching helps to keep your muscles long and supple and releases tension in your body and your mind.

Always stretch muscles that you have worked. Each strength exercise is accompanied by a complementary stretch recommendation so that you can stretch immediately after the exercise or you can combine a series of stretches to complete your training session. You will also find a mobility and flexibility program on page 182 for when you really want to stretch out your body and settle your soul.

Stretching tips

- Take the stretch to the point of slight tightness. Hold it there and breathe naturally for 40 to 60 seconds.
- Move a little further into the stretch if you feel the muscle relax and release.
- Discomfort and shaking are both signs of pushing your stretches too far.

Stretch and relax

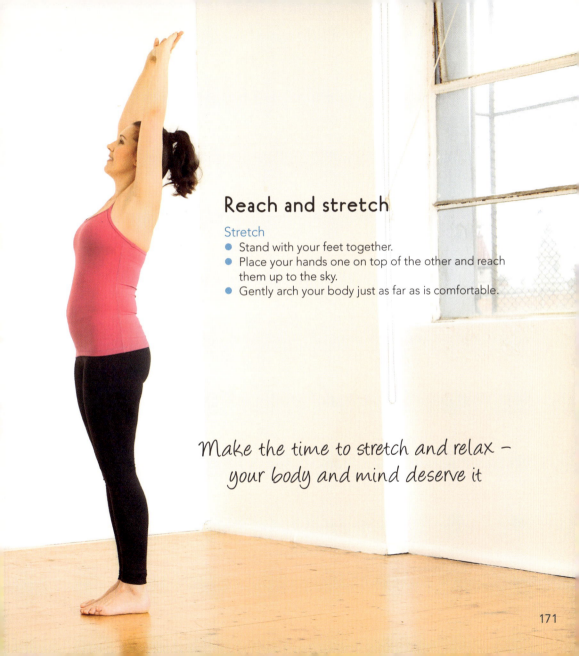

Reach and stretch

Stretch
- Stand with your feet together.
- Place your hands one on top of the other and reach them up to the sky.
- Gently arch your body just as far as is comfortable.

Make the time to stretch and relax – your body and mind deserve it

Stretches

Triceps stretch

- Reach your right arm up beside your ear.
- Bend your elbow to place your hand behind your neck.
- Use your left hand to gently push down on your right elbow until your feel a slight stretch at the back of your arm.
- After 10 slow breaths then repeat with the other arm.

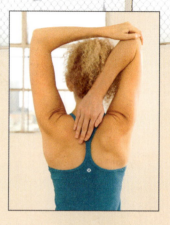

Chest stretch

- Stand side-on to the wall, with your hand on the wall slightly below shoulder height.
- Turn away from the wall to feel a stretch across your chest and shoulder.
- Hold the stretch for 10 slow breaths then change sides.

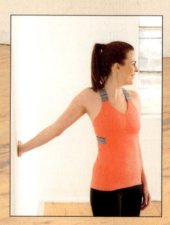

Upper-back stretch

- With one hand over the other reach your arms in front of you at shoulder height.
- Gently push your arms forwards.
- Feel your shoulder blades gliding forwards.
- Tilt your head downwards and round your upper back.
- Hold for 10 slow breaths.

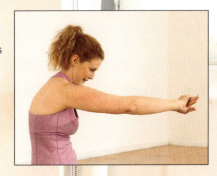

Hip-flexor stretch

- Take a big step back with your right foot.
- Place the ball of your foot on the floor but keep your heel up.
- Bend your left knee to lunge forwards.
- Push your right thigh forwards to feel a stretch across the front of your hip.
- Reach your hands back behind you to add a chest stretch.
- Hold for 10 slow breaths before changing legs.

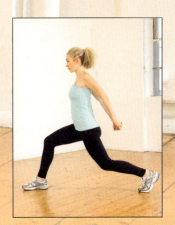

Supine rotation

- Lie on your back with your knees bent.
- Extend your arms to the side.
- Keeping your feet and knees together roll your knees to one side and look the other way.
- Hold the stretch for 10 slow breaths then, keeping your feet on the floor, slowly change sides.

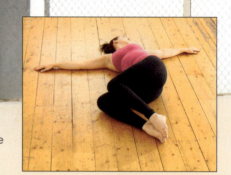

Seated hamstring stretch

- Sit on the floor with one leg extended in front of you.
- Keeping your back straight lean down the extended leg until you feel a stretch behind your thigh.
- Hold for 10 slow breaths then change legs.

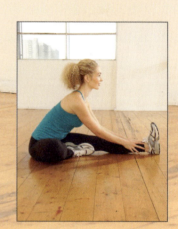

Kneeling back-and-butt stretch

- Kneel on the floor with your hands out in front of you.
- Sit back on your heels and stretch your arms forwards to stretch your back, butt and arms.

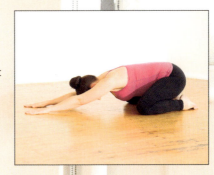

Side stretch

- Sit on ball or stand with your feet wide.
- Roll across to one side.
- Reach your arm by your ear to feel a long stretch through your arm and side.
- Support your body on your thigh through the other arm.

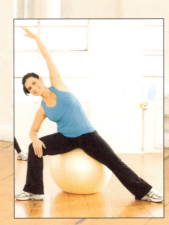

Prone quads stretch

- Lie on your front.
- Bring one foot up behind you.
- Hold your foot by the ankle and gently pull it towards your bottom.
- Hold for 10 slow breaths then repeat on the other leg.

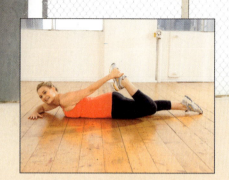

Supine hamstring stretch

- Lie on your back with both knees bent.
- Raise one leg towards the ceiling and hold it with both hands behind your thigh.
- Gently draw your leg towards you until you feel a slight stretch down the back of your thigh.
- Keep your tail bone and head on the floor.
- Hold for 10 slow breaths then change legs.

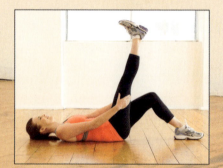

Supine gluteals stretch

- Lie on your back with both knees bent.
- Cross your right foot over your left thigh.
- Put your right hand through the hole and your left hand around the outside of your left leg to hold your left shin.
- Gently pull towards you to feel a stretch in your right buttock.
- Hold for 10 breaths, uncross and change legs.

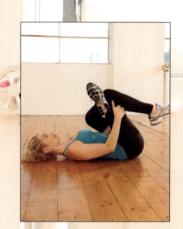

Prone extension

- Lie on your front with your hands under your shoulders.
- Prop yourself on your elbows and hold yourself here.
- If your back feels comfortable push through your hands to lift and extend a little further.
- Hold the position where you feel a slight stretch. Relax then repeat.

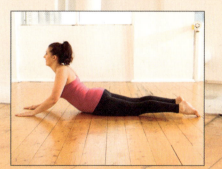

Listen to your body, progress gently, follow the program that's best for you

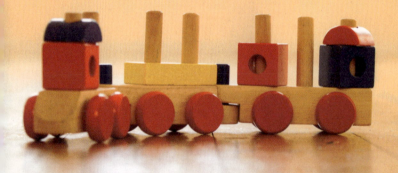

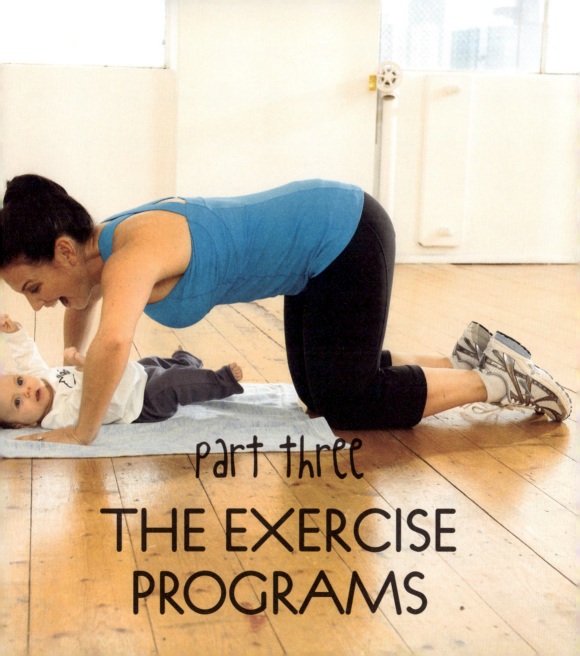

part three
THE EXERCISE PROGRAMS

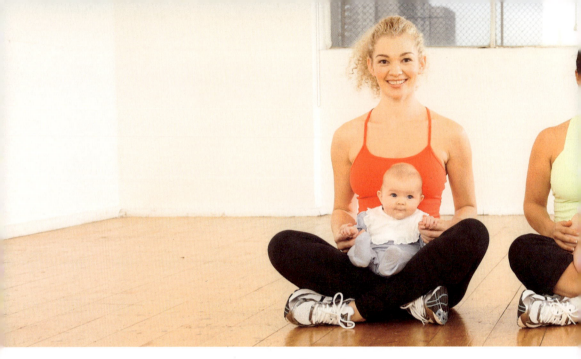

Exercise Programs

Combine the exercises in *Mums Shape Up* to create your own personalised postnatal fitness program or select from one of the following physiotherapy-designed programs according to your stage, fitness, lifestyle and goals. Programs vary in their intensity and style, providing options for women needing to take it easy after having their baby through to those who are well-recovered and ready to bridge the gap, progressing towards pre-pregnancy fitness regimes.

If finding time is your challenge or you want to lighten the load on your body you will enjoy the 10-minute programs that allow you to fit new-mum specific, safe and effective exercise into your day, every day.

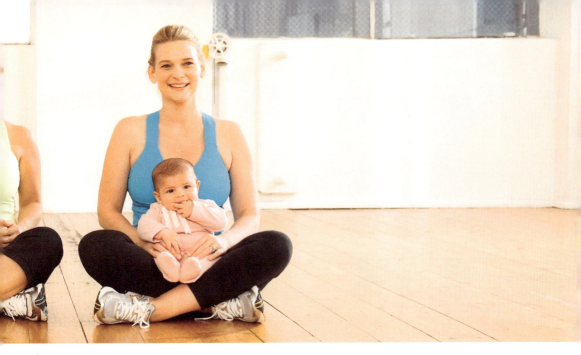

Program training tips

- Perform quality pelvic-floor exercises three times per day, alternating between long holds and quick lifts. Your pelvic-floor exercises within these programs can be long holds or quick lifts or a set of each.
- Aim to include time for relaxation daily, either after your exercise or at another time that is convenient.
- The exercises from 'Stroller fitness' and 'Mum-and-bub workout' sections can be followed as complete programs. (The exercises from these sections can also be included in other workouts without the baby or pram.)
- Always take the time to include the appropriate stretches and add extra mobility and flexibility moves to suit your body's needs.
- Listen to your body and check your posture frequently.

1 Early days

After your initial few days of rest and recovery (page 44) you will start to become more active, just from looking after and enjoying your baby. Starting out with gentle mobility and flexibility exercises will help keep your body free of tension.

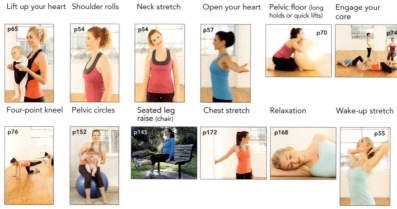

| Lift up your heart | Shoulder rolls | Neck stretch | Open your heart | Pelvic floor (long holds or quick lifts) | Engage your core |
| p65 | p54 | p54 | p57 | p70 | p74 |

| Four-point kneel | Pelvic circles | Seated leg raise (chair) | Chest stretch | Relaxation | Wake-up stretch |
| p76 | p152 | p145 | p172 | p168 | p55 |

2 Settling in

Enjoy gentle walking around the house, garden or out with your pram, plus a few strain-free exercises. Listen to your body and modify exercise to suit your specific stage of recovery.

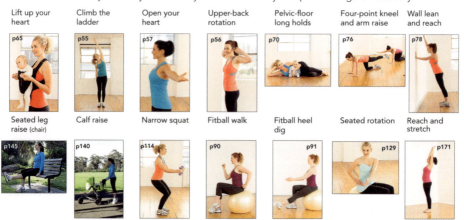

| Lift up your heart | Climb the ladder | Open your heart | Upper-back rotation | Pelvic-floor long holds | Four-point kneel and arm raise | Wall lean and reach |
| p65 | p55 | p57 | p56 | p70 | p76 | p78 |

| Seated leg raise (chair) | Calf raise | Narrow squat | Fitball walk | Fitball heel dig | Seated rotation | Reach and stretch |
| p145 | p140 | p114 | p90 | p91 | p129 | p171 |

3 Adding a touch of strength

As the weeks turn to months you can combine the following with a light walk or five to 10 minutes of low-impact exercises (page 88) if your body feels ready and able.

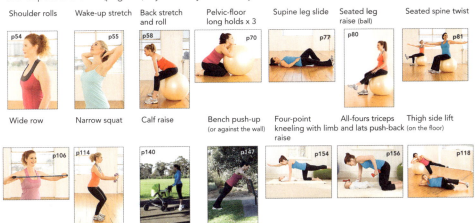

4 Posture: core and pelvic floor

A fabulous 'every other day' option to allow you to continue to prioritise inner strength as your overall fitness improves.

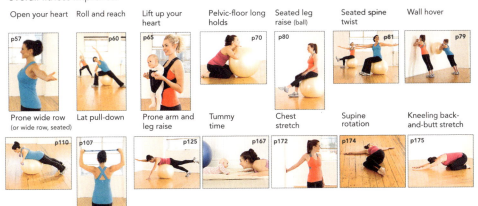

5 All-round shape-up 1

Follow 10 to 15 minutes' walking or another style of low-impact exercise that suits your body with this selection of strength options for a lighter level all-round-conditioning program. Remember to include recommended stretches for each strength move.

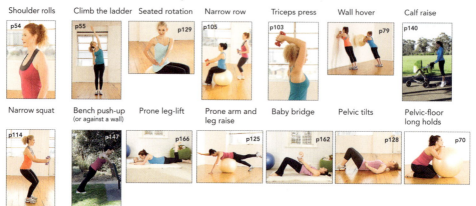

6 All-round shape-up 2

As you feel stronger inside and out, you can progress your strength program. Continue to listen to your body and put quality before quantity. Add the following to a brisk walk or 15 to 20 minutes of other cardio fitness, or perform it as a workout in its own right.

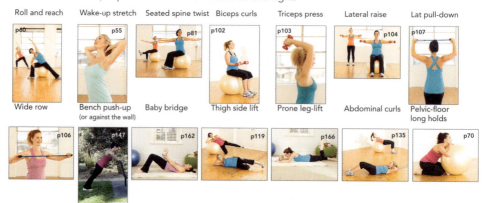

7 Fitball gentle
A gentler fitball training session uniting inner and outer strength.

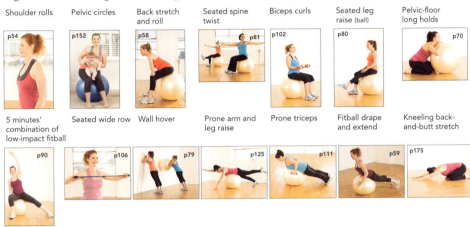

8 Fitball progressions
Get on the ball for a stronger workout once your body is well-recovered and looking for more.

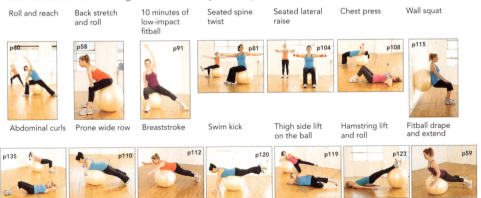

9 10-minute lower body, level 1

A straight and strong lower-body workout, making the best out of a 10-minute opportunity.

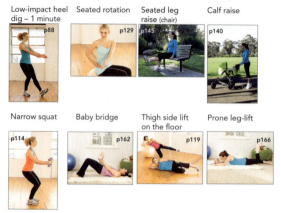

Low-impact heel dig – 1 minute p88
Seated rotation p129
Seated leg raise (chair) p145
Calf raise p140

Narrow squat p114
Baby bridge p162
Thigh side lift on the floor p119
Prone leg-lift p166

10 10-minute lower body, level 2

Progressions for toning below the belt.

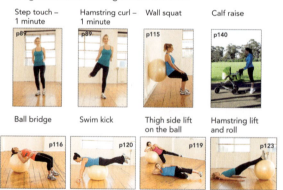

Step touch – 1 minute p89
Hamstring curl – 1 minute p89
Wall squat p115
Calf raise p140

Ball bridge p116
Swim kick p120
Thigh side lift on the ball p119
Hamstring lift and roll p123

11 10-minute upper body
Tone and strengthen your upper body when time is short.

Shoulder rolls p54

Climb the ladder p55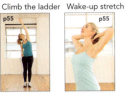

Wake-up stretch p55

Biceps curls p102

Triceps press p103

Lateral raise p104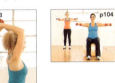

Narrow row p105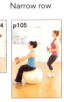

Bench push-up (or against the wall) p147

12 10-minute abs, back and butt, level 1
Focusing on your midsection without straining your back or pelvic floor.

Open your heart p57

Seated spine twist p81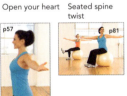

Lat pull-down p107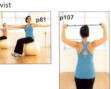

Wall lean and reach p78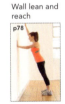

Prone arm and leg raise p125

All-fours triceps and lats push-back p156

Supine leg slide p77

Pelvic tilt p128

13 10-minute abs, back and butt, level 2

A stronger workout for your torso, when your body says you're ready.

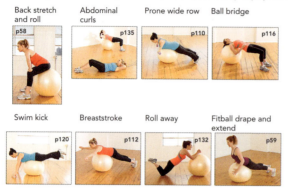

Back stretch and roll — p58
Abdominal curls — p135
Prone wide row — p110
Ball bridge — p116
Swim kick — p120
Breaststroke — p112
Roll away — p132
Fitball drape and extend — p59

14 Stretch and relax

Ease away the tension in your body and your mind.

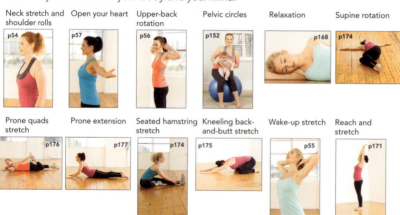

Neck stretch and shoulder rolls — p54
Open your heart — p57
Upper-back rotation — p56
Pelvic circles — p152
Relaxation — p168
Supine rotation — p174
Prone quads stretch — p176
Prone extension — p177
Seated hamstring stretch — p174
Kneeling back-and-butt stretch — p175
Wake-up stretch — p55
Reach and stretch — p171

Thank You

There are a number of wonderful people who have inspired and supported me in the creation of *Mums Shape Up*. Thank you to the fabulous team at Hachette, especially Kate Ballard, for your incredible patience, unfailing positive attitude, superb editing and for allowing me to share in decisions as we went along. Bronwyn Kidd, your photography is stunning and you are an absolute delight to work with. Thank you once again for your ingenious magic behind the lens. Thank you to designer Jude Rowe for your creative flair and finesse. Thank you to three friends and physiotherapists, Janetta Webb, Shira Kramer and Dianne Edmonds, for generously and happily sharing your time, advice and inspiration. A big thank you to Stef for your sensational production skills, tireless advice, cheerful encouragement and friendship. To the precious and incredibly photogenic mother-and-baby teams, thank you for your beautiful smiles and encouragement: Lauren and Allira, Lee and Jamie, Marie and Ines, Bree and Isla, Cassie and Parker, and Jess and Quinn.

To Alexie, Zoe and everyone at Lululemon Athletica Australia, I am grateful for your ongoing support and for dressing these new mums in their gorgeous exercise gear. Annette, of Gaia Organic Cotton, thank you so much for dressing our babies in such divine outfits. Thank you also to Meagan at Brooks Sports for the footwear.

Thank you to Kris at the White Space Photographic Studio and to Ziva for again allowing us to take photos in her beautiful home. To all the beautiful new mums out there, thank you for inspiring this book. To my mum and to all my immediate and extended family, thank you, just for being you.

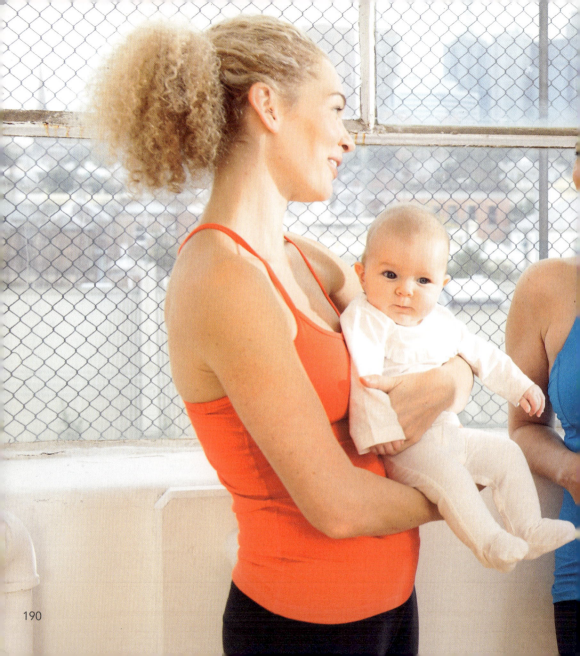

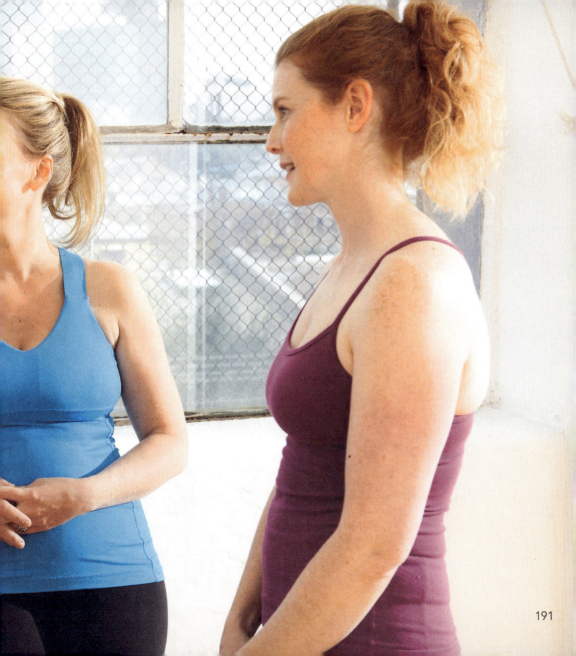

About the author

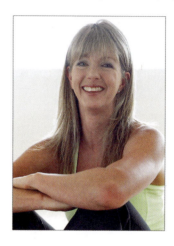

Lisa Westlake is a mother of two, a physiotherapist, a highly regarded fitness instructor and an international presenter. She lectures in several Melbourne universities and is involved in promoting community health and well-being through her writing, ABC Radio health and fitness segments and hosting community events such as the Mother's Day Classic and Run Melbourne. Through her business, Physical Best, Lisa combines her knowledge and skills in both physiotherapy and fitness to provide exercise programs for people of all ages and abilities. Alongside her passion for helping women achieve their physical and emotional best, Lisa has drawn on over 20 years' experience of instructing pre- and postnatal fitness classes to bring a wealth of knowledge and information to *Exercising for Two* and *Mums Shape Up*. Lisa has produced six fitness DVDs and has presented in numerous countries on all things health and fitness. Her first two books, *Strong to the Core* and *Strong and Stable* have been published in many countries. Lisa was awarded Australian Fitness Instructor of the Year in 2000, Australian Fitness Presenter of the Year in 2003 and Australian Fitness Author of the Year in 2009.

www.physicalbest.com